POCKET

EMERGENT   SERIOUS ADVERSE EVENTS IN PSYCHOPHARMACOLOGY

Edited by

Richard Balon, M.D.
Mary K. Morreale, M.D.

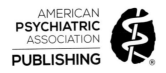

AMERICAN
PSYCHIATRIC
ASSOCIATION
PUBLISHING ®

If you wish to buy 50 or more copies of the same title, please go to www.appi.org/specialdiscounts for more information.

Copyright © 2023 American Psychiatric Association Publishing

ALL RIGHTS RESERVED

First Edition

Manufactured in the United States of America on acid-free paper

27   26   25   24   23   5   4   3   2   1

ISBN 978-1-61537-453-3 (paperback), 978-1-61537-454-0 (ebook)

American Psychiatric Association Publishing
800 Maine Avenue SW, Suite 900
Washington, DC 20024-2812
www.appi.org

Library of Congress Cataloging-in-Publication Data
A CIP record is available from the Library of Congress.

British Library Cataloguing in Publication Data
A CIP record is available from the British Library.

Contents

Contributors ix

Introduction xv

1 Acute Dystonia 1

    Bhargav Patel, M.D.
    Urja Shah, M.A.
    Nagy A. Youssef, M.D., Ph.D.

2 Agitation 11

    Jeffrey J. Rakofsky, M.D.

3 Agranulocytosis With Clozapine and
Other Psychotropic Medications 21

    Obiora Onwuameze, M.D., Ph.D.
    Eric Black, M.D.

4 Benzodiazepines in Combination With
Opioids: Therapeutic Benefit Versus
Fatal Overdose 29

    Edward Silberman, M.D.

5 Cardiac Emergencies Such as
Arrhythmias, QTc Prolongation, and
Cardiomyopathy 39

    Margo C. Funk, M.D., M.A.
    Junyang Lou, M.D., Ph.D.

6 Discontinuation of
Psychotropic Medications 51

    Vladan Starcevic, M.D., Ph.D., FRANZCP

7 Hepatotoxicity of
Psychotropic Medications 63

Ashika Bains, M.D.

8 Hypertensive Crisis Associated With
Monoamine Oxidase Inhibitors 75

Mary K. Morreale, M.D.

9 Hyponatremia, Especially in
Older Adults 81

Art Walaszek, M.D.

10 Neuroleptic Malignant Syndrome 91

Michael Maksimowski, M.D.

11 Ocular Side Effects of
Psychotropic Medications 99

Haoxing Chen, M.D.
Richard Balon, M.D.

12 Overdoses of Psychotropic Medications
ANTIDEPRESSANTS, LITHIUM, AND
ANTIPSYCHOTICS 111

*Spencer Greene, M.D., M.S., FACEP, FACMT,
FAACT, FAAEM*

13 Polypharmacy and
Acute Side Effects 125

Sweta Bhoopatiraju, B.S.
Marissa Hirsch, M.D.
Harjinderpal Singh, B.S., B.Ed.
George Grossberg, M.D.

14 Pregnancy and Use of
Psychotropic Medication 135

Katherine Taljan, M.D.
Adele C. Viguera, M.D., M.P.H.

15 Seizure Risk Management 147

Nicholas A. Mischel, M.D., Ph.D.

16 Serotonin Syndrome 157

Memphis Diaz Garcia, M.D.
Rashi Aggarwal, M.D.

17 Substances With Addictive Potential
and Psychotropic Medications 167

Peter J. Na, M.D., M.P.H.
Sanya Virani, M.D., M.P.H.
Oluwole Jegede, M.D., M.P.H.
Adrienne Hicks, M.D., Ph.D.
Sivabalaji Kaliamurthy, M.D.
Aaron Wolfgang, M.D.
Ellen L. Edens, M.D.

18 Tardive Dyskinesia 181

Michael D. Jibson, M.D., Ph.D.

Index 193

POCKET GUIDE TO
EMERGENT AND SERIOUS ADVERSE EVENTS IN PSYCHOPHARMACOLOGY

Contributors

Rashi Aggarwal, M.D.
Vice-Chair and Residency Program Director; and Professor, Department of Psychiatry, Rutgers New Jersey Medical School, Newark, New Jersey

Ashika Bains, M.D.
Physician, Department of Psychiatry, Massachusetts General Hospital; and Instructor, Department of Psychiatry, Harvard Medical School, Boston, Massachusetts

Richard Balon, M.D.
Professor of Psychiatry and Anesthesiology; Associate Chair for Education and Faculty Affairs; and Program Director, Department of Psychiatry and Behavioral Neurosciences, Wayne State University School of Medicine, Detroit, Michigan

Sweta Bhoopatiraju, B.S.
Student, Department of Psychiatry and Behavioral Neuroscience, Saint Louis University School of Medicine, St. Louis, Missouri

Eric Black, M.D.
Assistant Professor, Department of Psychiatry, Southern Illinois University School of Medicine, Springfield, Illinois

Haoxing Chen, M.D.
Glaucoma Fellow, Kresge Eye Institute and Department of Ophthalmology, Visual and Anatomical Sciences, Wayne State University, Detroit, Michigan

Ellen L. Edens, M.D.
Associate Professor of Psychiatry, Yale School of Medicine, New Haven, Connecticut; and Substance Use Disorder Lead, National Telemental Health Center, VA Connecticut Healthcare System, West Haven, Connecticut

Margo C. Funk, M.D., M.A.
Vice Chair for Education, Director of Residency Education, and Director of Cardiovascular Psychiatry, Department of

Psychiatry, Brigham and Women's Hospital; Assistant Professor of Psychiatry, Department of Psychiatry, Harvard Medical School, Boston, Massachusetts

Memphis Diaz Garcia, M.D.
Resident, Department of Psychiatry, Rutgers New Jersey Medical School, Newark, New Jersey

Spencer Greene, M.D., M.S., FACEP, FACMT, FAACT, FAAEM
Director of Toxicology, Department of Emergency Medicine, HCA Houston Healthcare Kingwood; and Clinical Professor, University of Houston College of Medicine, Houston, Texas

George Grossberg, M.D.
Samuel W. Fordyce Professor, Department of Psychiatry and Behavioral Neuroscience, Saint Louis University School of Medicine, St. Louis, Missouri

Adrienne Hicks, M.D., Ph.D.
Assistant Professor of Clinical Psychiatry, Yale School of Medicine, New Haven, Connecticut; and Addiction Psychiatrist, VA Connecticut Healthcare System, West Haven, Connecticut

Marissa Hirsch, M.D.
Resident Psychiatrist, Department of Psychiatry and Behavioral Neuroscience, Saint Louis University School of Medicine, St. Louis, Missouri

Oluwole Jegede, M.D., M.P.H.
Assistant Professor of Psychiatry, Yale School of Medicine, New Haven, Connecticut; and Addiction Psychiatrist, Connecticut Mental Health Center, New Haven, Connecticut

Michael D. Jibson, M.D., Ph.D.
Professor of Psychiatry, University of Michigan, Ann Arbor, Michigan

Sivabalaji Kaliamurthy, M.D.
Attending Physician, Division of Psychiatry and Behavioral Sciences, Children's National Hospital, Washington, D.C.; Assistant Professor of Psychiatry, Howard University Col-

lege of Medicine, Washington, D.C.; and Instructor of Psychiatry, Yale School of Medicine, New Haven, Connecticut

Junyang Lou, M.D., Ph.D.
Interventional Cardiologist, Division of Cardiovascular Medicine, Brigham and Women's Hospital; Instructor of Medicine, Department of Medicine, Harvard Medical School, Boston, Massachusetts

Michael Maksimowski, M.D.
Assistant Clinical Professor, Department of Psychiatry, Wayne State University; and Staff Psychiatrist, John D. Dingell Veterans Affairs Medical Center, Detroit, Michigan

Nicholas A. Mischel, M.D., Ph.D.
Assistant Professor, Department of Psychiatry and Behavioral Neurosciences, Wayne State University School of Medicine, Detroit, Michigan

Mary K. Morreale, M.D.
Professor, Department of Psychiatry, Wayne State University, Detroit, Michigan

Peter J. Na, M.D., M.P.H.
Assistant Professor of Psychiatry, Yale School of Medicine, New Haven, Connecticut; and Addiction Psychiatrist, VA Connecticut Healthcare System, West Haven, Connecticut

Obiora Onwuameze, M.D., Ph.D.
Associate Professor and Director Clerkship, Department of Psychiatry, Southern Illinois University School of Medicine, Springfield, Illinois

Bhargav Patel, M.D.
Resident Physician, Department of Psychiatry and Health Behavior, Medical College of Georgia, Augusta, Georgia

Jeffrey J. Rakofsky, M.D.
Associate Professor and Director of Medical Student Education, Department of Psychiatry and Behavioral Sciences, Emory University School of Medicine, Atlanta, Georgia

Urja Shah, M.A.
D.O. Candidate, Campbell University School of Osteopathic Medicine, Buies Creek, North Carolina

Edward Silberman, M.D.
Professor of Psychiatry, Tufts Medical Center/Tufts University School of Medicine, Boston, Massachusetts

Harjinderpal Singh, B.S., B.Ed.
Student, Department of Psychiatry and Behavioral Neuroscience, Saint Louis University School of Medicine, St. Louis, Missouri

Vladan Starcevic, M.D., Ph.D., FRANZCP
Professor, Nepean Clinical School, Sydney Medical School, Faculty of Medicine and Health, University of Sydney, Sydney, Australia

Katherine Taljan, M.D.
Associate Staff, Psychiatry, Cleveland Clinic, Cleveland, Ohio

Adele C. Viguera, M.D., M.P.H.
Clerkship Director of Psychiatry and Staff Psychiatrist, Consultation Liaison Service, Cleveland Clinic, Cleveland, Ohio

Sanya Virani, M.D., M.P.H.
Director, Addiction Services, Worcester Recovery Center and Hospital, Worcester, Massachusetts; and Assistant Professor and Associate Program Director, Addiction Psychiatry Fellowship, University of Massachusetts Chan Medical School, Worcester, Massachusetts

Art Walaszek, M.D.
Professor of Psychiatry and Medicine, University of Wisconsin School of Medicine and Public Health, Madison, Wisconsin

Aaron Wolfgang, M.D.
Assistant Professor, Uniformed Services University, Bethesda, Maryland; and Adjunct Assistant Professor of Psychiatry, Yale School of Medicine, New Haven, Connecticut

Nagy A. Youssef, M.D., Ph.D.
Director of Clinical Research, Director of ECT Program, and Professor of Psychiatry, The Ohio State University College of Medicine, Wexner Medical Center, Department of Psychiatry & Behavioral Health, Harding Hospital, Columbus, Ohio

Disclosures

The following contributor to this book has indicated a financial interest in or other affiliation with a commercial supporter, a manufacturer of a commercial product, a provider of a commercial service, a nongovernmental organization, and/or a government agency, as listed below:

Margo C. Funk, M.D., M.A., has received a speaking honorarium of less than $1,000 from Acadia Pharmaceuticals for a 4-hour Education Session for Scientific Team on QTc Prolongation (July 2021).

Introduction

The Art of Prescribing and Surviving Emergent and Serious Side Effects in Psychopharmacology

Most psychotropic medications are fairly safe when prescribed appropriately. However, like other medications, psychotropic medications are associated with various side effects. Although some of them are rare and paradoxical, others are quite common and even expected. Although most associated side effects are mild and require no intervention other than cautiously waiting to see whether they subside, sometimes dose adjustment or the addition of another medication is necessary.

The focus of this pocket guide is on those adverse effects that we, in consultation with our colleagues, considered to be serious and potentially life-threatening. The chapters, authored by a combination of experts and novices in the field, provide summaries of the current state of knowledge on particular topics and are not simply opinions based on personal experience.

We conceptualized this pocket guide as a simple and practical reference book with chapters listed in alphabetical order. The information contained is up to date (e.g., the management of hypertensive crisis with monoamine oxidase inhibitors). We strove to keep the structure of chapters cohesive, with an introduction followed by sections on recognition and detection, culprit medications, assessment, management, and follow-up management. The user can easily navigate through the text, choosing to read it in its entirety or to skip some chapters or section(s) when a quick decision is needed. However, this book is intended to be read and used as a whole because we believe that the information contained within is necessary for a comprehensive understanding of prescribing in psychiatry.

This pocket guide is intended to be what it is, a pocket guide. It does not cover all side effects like some complete volumes on this topic—for instance, Goldberg and Ernst's (2019) book on managing side effects of psychotropic medications, which is an excellent reference text. Ours is a volume mostly for psychopharmacology beginners and is intended to be carried around and consulted when one suspects a serious side effect caused by a psychopharmacological agent and needs information on acute management and further steps.

The management of side effects, similar to clinical psychopharmacology itself, is at the crossroads of the art of prescribing and clinical and, at times, basic science. The art of prescribing, especially in the case of managing side effects, is not always supported by perfect evidence. Much of our knowledge about side-effect management comes from case reports and case series. It is understandable that there are few large, well-designed studies on side-effect management because there is often no effective way to investigate certain conditions (e.g., neuroleptic malignant syndrome). Given the lack of consistent evidence, managing side effects often involves the art of patient care.

As Glick et al. (2009) noted, "The art of psychopharmacology is found in the management of intricate situations that don't quite follow the practice guidelines, and it is this art that guides many of everyday decisions clinicians make" (p. 423). They list practical advice that is applicable to our pocket guide, such as the need to always warn patients about major side effects in addition to possible controversies regarding psychiatric medications in the media (many television commercials end their list of side effects with "and death") and the fact that not every problem that looks like a side effect is necessarily a side effect (which signifies the importance of differential diagnosis). Glick et al. (2009) emphasized the importance of frequent communication with patients and families through psychoeducation and recommended being available via various means of communication. Glick et al.'s (2009) final words tell us that the quality of psychopharmacology practice is based on a combination of knowledge, experience, judgment, and luck. In most clinical situations, diagnosis should precede the setting of goals, which should precede treatment. "How this is done—the process of managing treatment of patients and their families, often over the course of a lifetime—is in part the 'art of psychopharmacology'" (p. 423). We believe that these words apply to the assessment and management of the serious and emergent side effects covered in this pocket guide and that the information in this book will provide readers with important knowledge to improve patient care.

Richard Balon, M.D.

Mary K. Morreale, M.D.

References

Glick ID, Balon RJ, Ballon J, Rovine D: Teaching pearls from the lost art of psychopharmacology. J Psychiatr Pract 15(5):423–426, 2009 19820559

Goldberg JF, Ernst CL: Managing the Side Effects of Psychotropic Medications, 2nd Edition. Washington, DC, American Psychiatric Association Publishing, 2019

Chapter 1

Acute Dystonia

Bhargav Patel, M.D.
Urja Shah, M.A.
Nagy A. Youssef, M.D., Ph.D.

Acute dystonia can result from various medical conditions and medications; however, for the purpose of this chapter, we focus on psychotropic-induced acute dystonia. Dystonic reactions, or acute dystonia, are neurological movement disorders characterized by muscular rigidity or excessive muscle contractions of one or more muscle groups that lead to abnormal posturing or movements. The exact mechanism of action of acute dystonia is unknown but is postulated to be related to the dopaminergic and cholinergic systems in the basal ganglia and nigrostriatal pathways of the brain. Within the field of psychiatry, acute dystonia is most commonly seen as a side effect of antipsychotic medications. Antipsychotic medications are used most commonly to treat psychotic episodes and psychotic disorders and for their mood-stabilizing and antimanic properties. These medications are also used to treat delirium and acute aggression and as augmenting agents for depressive and anxiety disorders.

Dystonia can occur virtually anywhere in the body with varying manifestations. Symptoms are not always obvious, which can lead to under- and misdiagnosis. Associated muscle spasms can be sustained or intermittent.

Acute dystonic reactions can be induced by any dopamine D_2 receptor–blocking agent but are most commonly seen with antipsychotic and antiemetic medications. There is an infrequent association with the antidepressant citalopram (Moosavi et al. 2014). Because the occurrence of dystonic reactions varies from medication to medication, the overall incidence is not known. With metoclopramide and prochlorperazine, up to 1% of patients experience acute dystonia (Campbell 2001).

Acute dystonic reactions typically occur within the first week of initiating a dopamine-blocking medication. Data suggest that 50% of dystonic reactions happen within the first 48 hours of initiation of a new medication treatment or dose increase, and up to 90% of the reactions occur within the first 5 days (Kowalski 2020).

Acute dystonia can manifest in a diverse clinical manner with a wide variation in intensity and acuity. These reactions can be particularly uncomfortable and frightening for patients. If patients are not educated about dystonia as a potential side effect of medication treatment, the physician-patient relationship can be strained. In patients at high risk for dystonia, such as younger patients initiating a high-potency typical antipsychotic, prophylactic prevention with an anticholinergic medication should be considered. The most common dystonias occur in the head and neck region and manifest as torticollis, trismus, mouth-opening dystonias, grimaces, blepharospasms, difficulties swallowing, dysarthria, and oculogyric crises (see also Chapter 11, "Ocular Side Effects of Psychotropic Medications"). Other forms of dystonia include generalized dystonia involving many muscle groups across the body that can lead to opisthotonos (van Harten et al. 1999). Additional symptoms of dystonia include buccolingual crisis, tortipelvic crisis, and pseudomacroglossia, which are described in further detail later in the "Assessment" section (Campbell 2001). Rare life-threatening dystonias can occur when muscular spasms involve the laryngeal muscles, causing stridor, shortness of breath and potential airway compromise, and sudden death (van Harten et al. 1999).

Risk factors for acute dystonia are important to recognize. Most studies indicate that acute dystonia is more common in men than in women and in younger people compared with elderly people, with a linear decline of occurrence with age (van Harten et al. 1999). Younger age is one of the strongest risk factors for medication-induced dystonia following psychotropic use (Keepers and Casey 1987), and children between ages 12 and 19 years have the highest risk (van Harten et al. 1999). The incidence of dystonia in elderly people is low, which is thought to be due to a decline in dopamine receptor activity with age (Volkow et al. 1998). Although patients younger than 30 are more likely to have generalized dystonia, those older than 30 are more likely to have localized dystonic reactions (Cloud and Jinnah 2010). Males have about twice the relative risk of females for acute dystonic reactions to antipsychotic medications, yet there appear to be only minor correlations with the dose and the potency of dopamine-blocking medications (Keepers and Casey 1987). The greatest risk factor for a dystonic reaction is a history of acute dystonia related to medication use, with up to six times increased relative risk (Keepers and Casey 1987). Other risk factors include recent cocaine use, hypocalcemia, hypoparathyroidism (which can cause hypocalcemia), and dehydration (van Harten et al. 1999).

Although the exact cause of medication-induced acute dystonia is not known, the mechanism of action is thought to be related to the ratio of dopamine to acetylcholine blockade in the basal ganglia (van Harten et al. 1999). High-potency antipsychotic agents such as haloperidol, fluphenazine, and pimozide have a higher degree of D_2 receptor blockade compared with anticholinergic activity and are therefore associated with a greater risk for acute dystonia. Conversely, low-potency antipsychotic medications (e.g., chlorpromazine), which have a lower ratio of dopamine to acetylcholine blockade, have decreased incidence of dystonic reactions (van Harten et al. 1999). The efficacy of anticholinergic medications in the treatment of dystonia is thought to be related to altering this ratio. Atypical antipsychotic medications that are partial agonists of D_2 receptors have far less risk of dystonia when compared with typical antipsychotic agents.

Recognition and Detection

Patients experiencing acute dystonia typically present with involuntary, sustained or intermittent muscular contractions in one or more muscle groups within the first week (most commonly in the first 96 hours) of initiating a psychotropic agent or significantly increasing the dose. Although dystonia can occur in any muscle group in the body, the most common location is in the head and neck area.

Culprit Medications

As mentioned, acute dystonic reactions happen because of medications that block dopamine receptors, which include antipsychotics, antiemetics, and, rarely, certain antidepressants. Antipsychotics with strong dopamine blockade and high-potency antipsychotics have the highest risk of extrapyramidal symptoms such as acute dystonia. These include haloperidol, fluphenazine, paliperidone, and risperidone. The risk is relatively lower with ziprasidone, aripiprazole, olanzapine, and quetiapine but still exists for any antipsychotic except for clozapine, which extremely rarely causes dystonia. In terms of antiemetics, culprit medications include metoclopramide, and with respect to antidepressants, acute dystonic reactions can in rare cases be caused by citalopram.

Assessment

When a patient is being assessed for acute dystonic reactions, the history and physical examination are central. First, the patient should be asked whether an antipsychotic or a dopamine-blocking agent was recently introduced or increased in dose. Given the risk factors discussed earlier, the patient's age, sex, and history of acute dystonic reactions to medications should be considered. Other risk factors to assess are a history of hypocalcemia, cocaine use, hypoparathyroidism, and dehydration. Following the history, a physical examination should be performed, and the patient should be checked for signs of dystonia (if they are not readily obvious), which can be anywhere in the body and vary in manifestation. The primary way to assess dystonia is through visual observation. Because the most common locations are in the head and neck region, particular attention should be given to this area for signs of muscular contractions or rigidity. Unless there is significant suspicion of other causes of acute dystonia, laboratory tests and neuroimaging are not urgently needed.

Symptoms to pay attention to include spasm of extraorbital muscles with upward deviation (oculogyric crises, which are further discussed in Chapter 11); the head or neck being turned to one side (torticollis); painful neck extension (opisthotonos); a protruded and swollen-feeling tongue (pseudomacroglossia, which can be part of a buccolingual crisis); spasticity and contraction of the trunk muscles, abdominal wall, and hip and pelvis (tortipelvic crisis); an inability to open the mouth or jaw (trismus); slurred speech (dysarthria); and difficulty breathing (laryngospasm or pharyngeal spasms) (Campbell 2001). Signs of laryngospasm should be urgently addressed because this can be a life-threatening medical emergency. Although rare, spasm of the laryngeal muscles can cause sudden death, and immediate intubation may be necessary if it is severe.

Because dystonia can be associated with medical disease, the clinician should consider other potential causes and associated conditions depending on the clinical presentation. Disorders to consider include various inherited metabolic diseases and vitamin deficiencies as well as Wilson's disease and parkinsonism. Patients with these disorders, however, are most likely to present with chronic dystonia rather than the acute dystonias that occur within a few days of psychotropic medication initiation. The differential diagnoses of dystonia should also include pseudodystonia, psychogenic dystonia, catatonia, tardive dystonia, hypocalcemia, and temporal lobe epilepsies.

Pseudodystonia, as the name implies, describes a condition that mimics dystonia. Pseudodystonia is described as abnormal postures, repetitive movements, or both, for which the results of clinical, imaging, laboratory, or electrophysiological investigations are not compatible with dystonia. Potential causes of pseudodystonia include nonneurological disorders of the musculoskeletal system (subluxation of joints, joint deformities, congenital torticollis), disorders of sensory pathways (parietal lobe damage, neuropathy), disorders of motor pathways (stiff person syndrome, myoclonic disorders), and compensatory postures in other neurological disorders (head tilt due to vestibulopathy) (Berlot et al. 2019).

Psychogenic dystonia, like conversion disorders, can occur acutely and can be confused for acute dystonia. Although no one symptom can unambiguously distinguish psychogenic dystonia from an organic dystonia, psychogenic dystonia should be considered when symptoms occur after an acute stressor and improve when the patient believes that they are not being observed. It is important to note that organic dystonic reactions can worsen with fear and improve with relaxation; thus, these phenomena should not be used as proof of a psychogenic etiology (van Harten et al. 1999).

Catatonia also can be confused for acute dystonia, but it is not temporally related to the initiation of psychotropic medications and has other associated symptoms such as mutism and akinesia. Unlike acute dystonia, tardive dystonia is an extrapyramidal side effect that occurs after months or years of psychotropic treatment, not days, and does not respond rapidly to anticholinergic treatment (van Harten et al. 1999). Temporal lobe epilepsies can also manifest with dystonic symptoms acutely but, again, will not be associated with the recent initiation or dose increase of an associated medication. If the patient does not respond to treatment with anticholinergics, which is discussed in the "Management" section, further workup can be initiated, such as checking calcium and parathyroid hormone levels, both of which can cause symptoms that look like dystonia and exacerbate existing dystonic reactions.

Management

Treatment of acute dystonia is simple and usually highly effective within a brief period. Treatment centers around balancing dopamine and acetylcholine within the brain and basal ganglia. The first step in treatment is administration of an anticholinergic agent or antihistaminergic medication with anticholinergic activity. Medications must have CNS penetration to have a benefit. Although intramuscular administration is most common, both intravenous and intramuscular routes of administration have a similar time of onset and action. Most patients will respond within 5 minutes and will be free of symptoms within 20 minutes. If the first dose fails, a second dose may be given after 30 minutes. If a second dose fails to effectively reduce symptoms, other diagnoses should be considered.

In the emergency department setting, the most commonly used medications for the treatment of acute dystonia are benztropine, an anticholinergic medication, and diphenhydramine, an antihistamine with significant anticholinergic activity. Both agents have significant CNS penetration and should resolve symptoms within 30 minutes. The dosing for benztropine in adults is 1–2 mg IM, whereas the dosing for diphenhydramine is 25–50 mg IM. Following an acute episode of dystonia, relapse prophylaxis with oral anticholinergic medications should continue for 4–7 days. In pediatric patients, the use of benztropine is considered off-label, and the dosing of diphenhydramine is 1 mg/kg (up to 50 mg) (Lewis and O'Day 2020). Anticholinergic side effects include dry mouth, dry eyes, constipation, blurred vision, urinary retention, confusion, and delirium. These symptoms, specifically confusion and delirium, have a significantly higher risk in elderly people, especially those with preexisting cognitive impairment.

Second-line therapy for acute dystonia includes the use of intramuscular or intravenous benzodiazepines, such as lorazepam and diazepam. In cases of oculogyric crises that do not respond to first-line treatments, clonazepam is effective (Horiguchi and Inami 1989).

In severe life-threatening cases of laryngeal dystonia in which respiratory compromise or stridor is present, intravenous administration of anticholinergics is strongly recommended. In addition, patients who present with respiratory symptoms may require supplemental oxygen, assisted ventilation, and intubation to protect the airway.

Following successful treatment, the offending medication should be either decreased in dose or discontinued, with consideration of an alternative medication with less risk for dystonia. Without medical treatment, most cases of acute dystonia resolve within 12–48 hours. However, because of the significant discomfort for the patient and the potential for future noncompliance with the medication regimen, dystonic reactions should be treated promptly. If the offending medication is continued, treatment with an anticholinergic medication should be considered to prevent relapse. In patients at high risk for psychotropic-induced acute dystonia, such as young patients between ages 12 and 19 years, particularly males, anticholinergic prophylaxis can be given to prevent an episode of acute dystonia along with the initiation of psychotropic medications (Arana et al. 1988; Spina et al. 1993).

Follow-Up Management

Following acute treatment, patients should be given benztropine 1–2 mg by mouth twice a day for up to 7 days to prevent recurrence. No long-term effects of acute dystonia are expected, especially if the triggering medication is discontinued.

Conclusion

Acute dystonia induced by psychotropic medication is most common in younger people, males, cocaine users, and those taking high-potency antipsychotic medications. It can affect any muscle group but is mostly found in the head and neck area. In most cases, acute dystonia is not life-threatening and can be treated easily with anticholinergic medications such as benztropine and diphenhydramine, and rapid resolution occurs within 5–20 minutes. It is important to be aware of life-threatening situations such as laryngeal and pharyngeal dystonia and to treat them appropriately.

Key Points

Acute dystonia induced by psychotropics is not uncommon with antipsychotic medication use, especially high-potency antipsychotic agents. Acute dystonia can also occur with antiemetics and, rarely, with antidepressants.

Acute dystonia manifests with sustained or intermittent muscle contractions in one or more muscle groups within several days of medication initiation or dose increase.

Fifty percent of cases of acute dystonia occur within the first 48 hours of medication initiation, and up to 90% occur within the first 5 days.

The exact mechanism of action of acute dystonia is unknown but is postulated to be related to the dopaminergic and cholinergic systems in the basal ganglia and nigrostriatal pathways of the brain.

The most common location of dystonia is the head and neck area.

Risk factors for dystonia include prior acute dystonic reaction, male sex, young age, cocaine use, hypocalcemia, hypoparathyroidism, and dehydration.

The most important risk factors for acute dystonia are a history of psychotropic medication use and a younger age (12–19 years).

Laryngeal dystonia is life-threatening and can manifest with dysphonia and stridor. Laryngeal dystonia should be treated as a medical emergency with intravenous anticholinergics, oxygen, and intubation as needed.

Acute dystonia is treated with anticholinergic medications, such as intramuscular benztropine and diphenhydramine.

Following an acute episode of dystonia, relapse prophylaxis with oral anticholinergic medications should continue for 4–7 days.

Anticholinergic side effects include dry mouth, dry eyes, constipation, blurred vision, urinary retention, confusion, and delirium.

References

Arana GW, Goff DC, Baldessarini RJ, Keepers GA: Efficacy of anticholinergic prophylaxis for neuroleptic-induced acute dystonia. Am J Psychiatry 145(8):993–996, 1988 2899403

Berlot R, Bhatia KP, Kojović M: Pseudodystonia: a new perspective on an old phenomenon. Parkinsonism Relat Disord 62:44–50, 2019 30819557

Campbell D: The management of acute dystonic reactions. Aust Prescr 24(1):19–20, 2001

Cloud LJ, Jinnah HA: Treatment strategies for dystonia. Expert Opin Pharmacother 11(1):5–15, 2010 20001425

Horiguchi J, Inami Y: Effect of clonazepam on neuroleptic-induced oculogyric crisis. Acta Psychiatr Scand 80(5):521–523, 1989 2574529

Keepers GA, Casey DE: Prediction of neuroleptic-induced dystonia. J Clin Psychopharmacol 7(5):342–345, 1987 2890672

Kowalski M: Medication-induced dystonic reactions clinical presentation: history, physical, causes. Medscape, 2020. Available at: https://emedicine.medscape.com/article/814632-clinical. Accessed April 20, 2021.

Lewis K, O'Day CS: Dystonic reactions. StatPearls, November 19, 2020. Available at: www.ncbi.nlm.nih.gov/books/NBK531466. Accessed January 4, 2021.

Moosavi SM, Ahmadi M, Monajemi MB: Acute dystonia due to citalopram treatment: a case series. Glob J Health Sci 6(6):295–299, 2014 25363102

Spina E, Sturiale V, Valvo S, et al: Prevalence of acute dystonic reactions associated with neuroleptic treatment with and without anticholinergic prophylaxis. Int Clin Psychopharmacol 8(1):21–24, 1993 8097213

van Harten PN, Hoek HW, Kahn RS: Acute dystonia induced by drug treatment. BMJ 319(7210):623–626, 1999 10473482

Volkow ND, Gur RC, Wang GJ, et al: Association between decline in brain dopamine activity with age and cognitive and motor impairment in healthy individuals. Am J Psychiatry 155(3):344–349, 1998 9501743

Chapter 2

Agitation

Jeffrey J. Rakofsky, M.D.

Psychomotor agitation describes physical and mental overactivity that is nonproductive and is associated with inner turmoil (Sadock et al. 2019). *Agitation* is the term the lay public often uses to describe irritability, which is the tendency to become easily annoyed and provoked to anger (Sadock et al. 2019). Although irritability and psychomotor agitation can occur simultaneously, they are different clinical phenomena. Psychomotor agitation can be seen across many psychiatric illnesses and is also a side effect of various medications, resulting from some physiological change induced by the medicine or a symptom of a syndrome caused by that medication. As such, it would be difficult to give the prevalence rates of psychomotor agitation without identifying the prevalence for all syndromes for which agitation could be an accompanying symptom. Here, causes of medication-induced psychomotor agitation are described and are categorized by class of psychotropic medication.

Recognition and Detection

Patients may describe psychomotor agitation as a need to move around, a feeling of restlessness, an inability to sit still, or the feeling that there is a motor driving them. Depending on the severity, some of their behaviors might include pacing around the room, tapping their feet, fidgeting with their hands, facial grimacing, picking at their nails or skin, and pulling their hair.

Culprit Medications

Antidepressants

Antidepressants include selective serotonin reuptake inhibitors (SSRIs), serotonin-norepinephrine reuptake inhibitors

(SNRIs), atypical antidepressants, tricyclic antidepressants (TCAs), and monoamine oxidase inhibitors (MAOIs). Psychomotor agitation can be seen with the increased anxiety associated with the initiation of antidepressants. Anxiety can lead to restlessness, taking the form of fidgeting or pacing. Anxiety associated with the initiation of antidepressants often resolves after a week or so of treatment and is thought to be mediated by an eventual downregulation of serotonin type 2C (5-HT$_{2C}$) receptors (Marcinkiewcz et al. 2016). The exception to this rule is anxiety associated with bupropion, a medication with very little serotonergic activity but with noradrenergic and dopaminergic activity. Psychomotor agitation also can be associated with manic or mixed-episode induction along with changes in mood, energy, confidence, and judgment. The risk of developing an antidepressant-induced manic or mixed episode is greatest in those with bipolar disorder who are taking SNRIs and TCAs and lowest among those taking SSRIs or MAOIs (Salvadore et al. 2010). Psychomotor agitation can develop in the setting of serotonin syndrome, which occurs when there is an excess of central and peripheral serotonin neurotransmission at various serotonin receptors as a result of high doses or polypharmacy with serotonergic medications. As part of this syndrome, patients may develop symptoms such as confusion, diaphoresis, diarrhea, hyperreflexia, tremor, shivering, and myoclonus, along with agitation (Ables and Nagubilli 2010).

Some antidepressants can lead to hyponatremia and resultant delirium. Psychomotor agitation is often a symptom of delirium. The risk for antidepressant-induced hyponatremia tends to be greatest in older patients, those concurrently taking thiazide diuretics, and those taking SSRIs and SNRIs. The risk seems to be lowest with TCAs and atypical antidepressants, such as mirtazapine (De Picker et al. 2014). Finally, another cause of psychomotor agitation associated with antidepressant medications is anticholinergic toxicity, which can also lead to delirium. This toxicity is more likely to occur in those taking TCAs, which have significant anticholinergic properties relative to the other classes of antidepressants (Tune 2001).

Antipsychotics

Antipsychotics include first-generation agents (FGAs) and second-generation agents (SGAs). Psychomotor agitation can occur when patients develop acute or tardive akathisia, an extrapyramidal symptom characterized by a need to move and an inner sense of restlessness. Acute or tardive akathisia most commonly occurs with the use of FGAs but can occur with SGAs as well, especially high-potency SGAs taken in high doses (Kumar and Sachdev 2009). Although acute akathisia tends to develop within hours to days after drug initiation or dose increase, tardive akathisia develops at least 3 months after drug initiation or dose changes. In addition, agitation can occur after drug withdrawal and can include choreoathetoid limb and orofacial dyskinesias (Bratti et al. 2007).

Psychomotor agitation can also occur in the setting of tardive dyskinesia. Tardive dyskinesia results when chronic dopamine receptor blockade leads to supersensitivity of downstream dopamine D_2 receptor activity or an upregulation of D_2 receptors occurs. This leads to the development of involuntary, purposeless movements usually of the facial-oral muscles but of the limbs as well. Risk factors for developing tardive dyskinesia include age, race, neuroleptic dose, and years of previous exposure, and the 5-year incidence risk is 20% (Morgenstern and Glazer 1993).

Psychomotor agitation can also occur in the context of neuroleptic malignant syndrome (NMS), which consists of hyperthermia, muscle rigidity, autonomic instability, creatine phosphokinase elevation, myoglobinuria, leukocytosis, and metabolic acidosis. Risk factors include dehydration, elevated temperature, poor oral intake, agitation, high doses of neuroleptics, and history of NMS (Pelonero et al. 1998). Antipsychotics have been associated with catatonia, which at times can manifest with hyperactivity along with verbigeration, mutism, staring, grimacing, echolalia, and echopraxia.

Similar to antidepressants, antipsychotics can induce delirium via anticholinergic toxicity (Tune 2001). It would most likely occur with low-potency FGAs, which have greater cholinergic receptor blockade than other FGAs and SGAs. Restless legs syndrome (RLS), a condition that causes uncomfortable sensations in the legs or a need to move them, usually in the late afternoon or nighttime, has been associated with antipsychotic use. Moving the legs or walking around tends to help (Aggarwal et al. 2015).

Mood Stabilizers

Mood stabilizers include lithium, valproate, carbamazepine, and lamotrigine. Lithium, like antipsychotic medications, has been associated with RLS (Terao et al. 1991). Patients taking lithium can develop hypothyroidism as a result of lithium's effect on thyroxine release from the thyroid gland. Additionally, lithium can cause hypercalcemia because of its effects on parathyroid gland receptors. Both hypothyroidism and hypercalcemia can be associated with psychomotor agitation. Lithium toxicity, which can occur when lithium levels exceed 1.2 mEq/L, can lead to confusion and psychomotor agitation. Lithium toxicity manifests with other signs of toxicity, including nausea, vomiting, tremulousness, and ataxia (Gitlin 2016). Both valproate and carbamazepine have been associated with hyperammonemia, leading to hyperammonemic encephalopathy and potentially psychomotor agitation. Among those taking valproate, the ammonia buildup is due to valproate's effects on the urea cycle. The cause associated with carbamazepine is unknown (Adams et al. 2009). Carbamazepine also has been associated with hyponatremia, which could lead to delirium.

Benzodiazepines and Nonbenzodiazepine Receptor Agonists

Benzodiazepines and nonbenzodiazepine receptor agonists have been associated with paradoxical agitation, named as such because there is a more common association with a reduction in physical movements by calming patients. Those at greatest risk for paradoxical agitation include children, elderly people, those with a genetic predisposition, those with a history of an alcohol use disorder, and those with psychological or psychiatric disturbances associated with anger or aggressive behavior (Mancuso et al. 2004). Benzodiazepine toxicity can also cause delirium and, therefore, psychomotor agitation. Finally, sleep-related activities (e.g., sleepwalking) induced by nonbenzodiazepine receptor agonists also can be associated with psychomotor agitation.

Miscellaneous Agents

Pramipexole is a partial D_2/D_3 agonist used as an adjunctive agent in the treatment of major depressive disorder and bipolar depression. It can induce a manic episode, which as described in the "Antidepressants" section, may include psychomotor agitation as a symptom. Stimulants, such as methylphenidate and amphetamines, used in the treatment of

ADHD and as an adjunctive agent in the treatment of depressive disorders also can induce manic and psychotic episodes, which can be associated with psychomotor agitation. In high doses, benztropine, an anticholinergic agent used to reduce extrapyramidal symptoms caused by antipsychotics, can lead to anticholinergic toxicity, delirium, and psychomotor agitation (Tune 2001). Psychomotor agitation can also develop as part of a withdrawal phenomenon from most of the medications listed in the various categories.

Assessment

As is often the case, the patient's history will be important to determine the nature of the underlying medication-induced psychomotor agitation. First and foremost, a temporal link must be made between the initiation or dose increase of the medication and the onset of the psychomotor agitation. The only exception to this rule is tardive akathisia and dyskinesia, which develop 3 months or longer after initiation or dose increase of a medication. If a temporal link is established, then questions about additional symptoms will help to further illuminate the underlying cause of the psychomotor agitation. For example, if the patient reports significant physical anxiety and/or an increase in uncontrollable worrying, then the agitation may stem from a medication-induced anxiety. However, in patients who report feeling joyful or irritable and simultaneously share ideas for new business opportunities and grandiose notions about themselves, the cause is likely a medication-induced manic episode.

Physical examination findings will be consistent with the syndromes associated with psychomotor agitation and induced by the medication. For example, NMS will likely manifest with lead-pipe rigidity. Serotonin syndrome will manifest with clonus and hyperreflexia. Lithium toxicity will manifest with significant tremors. Hyperammonemic encephalopathy will manifest with asterixis.

No laboratory studies are specific to psychomotor agitation, but there are studies that are specific to the cause of the agitation or syndromes induced by the medication. Examples include thyroid-stimulating hormone, calcium, and lithium levels for patients taking lithium; sodium levels for patients taking antidepressants and carbamazepine; iron levels for patients taking antipsychotics or lithium and experiencing

RLS symptoms; and ammonia levels for patients taking valproate and carbamazepine.

Rating scales of psychomotor agitation are primarily observational and can be used to characterize the nature and severity of the agitation or the associated syndrome. Those scales specific to agitation include the Pittsburgh Agitation Scale, the Overt Agitation Severity Scale, the Cohen-Mansfield Agitation Inventory Observational Tool, the Agitated Behavior Scale, and the Richmond Agitation-Sedation Scale. One of the main distinctions between these scales is the population of patients studied when the scales were developed. Other assessments are more indirect, focusing on the syndromes induced by the medications. Examples of such scales are the Young Mania Rating Scale for assessing manic symptoms, the Bush-Francis Catatonia Rating Scale for assessing catatonia severity, the Delirium Rating Scale for assessing delirium, and the Barnes Akathisia Rating Scale for measuring akathisia.

Management

Because of the numerous causes of medication-induced psychomotor agitation, it is beyond the scope of this chapter to identify all recommended treatments for all potential causes. Instead, the focus in this section is on the approach for managing medication-induced psychomotor agitation.

Although medications such as antipsychotics can be used to reduce agitation, it is best to first identify the cause and make that the target of treatment before adding unnecessary medications that may complicate the clinical picture. For example, antipsychotic-induced akathisia will become worse if the dose of the antipsychotic is increased to target the agitation rather than using evidence-based strategies to treat the akathisia. The same antipsychotic-induced worsening will occur in patients with NMS and catatonia. In some situations, it will be necessary to remove the underlying medication, and in other situations, it will be appropriate to continue that medication while either reducing the dose or adding another agent that addresses the cause of the psychomotor agitation. Continuing with the akathisia example, if the patient requires an antipsychotic for overall illness stability, it would be best to lower the dose or continue the antipsychotic at the current dose and consider adding a β-blocker, mirtazapine, or a benzodiazepine to target the akathisia. However, if the psychosis worsens with the lower dose and the akathisia does not improve with the use of additional agents or if the agitation leads to dangerous behaviors, then there would be cause to stop the antipsychotic and switch to one with weaker D_2 receptor binding.

The treatment setting for psychomotor agitation is a function of the associated dangerousness and the underlying syndrome caused by the medication. Medication-induced catatonia, mania, and delirium are best treated in a psychiatric inpatient unit, whereas medication-induced anxiety without suicidal thinking, hypomania, tardive dyskinesia, and RLS can be appropriately treated in an outpatient setting.

Follow-Up Management

Follow-up is required to ensure that the agitation is resolving, the psychiatric illness remains stable, and no intolerable side effects arise from any treatment added to address the agitation or the underlying syndrome associated with agitation. Patients receiving treatment in an outpatient setting should be seen weekly or less frequently depending on the severity of the psychomotor agitation. Follow-up telephone calls in between the patient's scheduled appointments can be made as well.

Conclusion

Psychomotor agitation is a symptom characterized by excessive movements and is associated with various syndromes caused by psychiatric medicines in every psychotropic class. History, physical examination, and laboratory studies can help identify the underlying cause of the psychomotor agitation or the associated syndrome. Assessment scales allow characterization of the nature and severity of the psychomotor agitation and/or the associated syndrome, depending on which scales are used. Management will necessitate either the removal of the underlying agent or the addition of an adjunct, allowing the patient to continue the inciting agent. The optimal strategy will depend on the dangerousness of the psychomotor agitation and the nature of the underlying cause.

Key Points

Psychomotor agitation describes an increase in motor and psychological activity and is not the same as irritability.

Except in the case of tardive akathisia and dyskinesia, a temporal link must be established to suggest that psychomotor agitation is caused by a psychotropic medication.

It is important to identify the underlying cause or syndrome associated with the psychomotor agitation and make that the target of treatment.

The decision to continue or stop the offending agent will be a function of the dangerousness of the agitation and the efficacy of adjunctive ameliorating agents.

References

Ables AZ, Nagubilli R: Prevention, recognition, and management of serotonin syndrome. Am Fam Physician 81(9):1139–1142, 2010 20433130

Adams EN, Marks A, Lizer MH: Carbamazepine-induced hyperammonemia. Am J Health Syst Pharm 66(16):1468–1470, 2009 19667003

Aggarwal S, Dodd S, Berk M: Restless leg syndrome associated with atypical antipsychotics: current status, pathophysiology, and clinical implications. Curr Drug Saf 10(2):98–105, 2015 24861990

Bratti IM, Kane JM, Marder SR: Chronic restlessness with antipsychotics. Am J Psychiatry 164(11):1648–1654, 2007 17974927

De Picker L, Van Den Eede F, Dumont G, et al: Antidepressants and the risk of hyponatremia: a class-by-class review of literature. Psychosomatics 55(6):536–547, 2014 25262043

Gitlin M: Lithium side effects and toxicity: prevalence and management strategies. Int J Bipolar Disord 4(1):27, 2016 27900734

Kumar R, Sachdev PS: Akathisia and second-generation antipsychotic drugs. Curr Opin Psychiatry 22(3):293–299, 2009 19378382

Mancuso CE, Tanzi MG, Gabay M: Paradoxical reactions to benzodiazepines: literature review and treatment options. Pharmacotherapy 24(9):1177–1185, 2004 15460178

Marcinkiewcz CA, Mazzone CM, D'Agostino G, et al: Serotonin engages an anxiety and fear-promoting circuit in the extended amygdala. Nature 537(7618):97–101, 2016 27556938

Morgenstern H, Glazer WM: Identifying risk factors for tardive dyskinesia among long-term outpatients maintained with neuroleptic medications: results of the Yale Tardive Dyskinesia Study. Arch Gen Psychiatry 50(9):723–733, 1993 8102845

Pelonero AL, Levenson JL, Pandurangi AK: Neuroleptic malignant syndrome: a review. Psychiatr Serv 49(9):1163–1172, 1998 9735957

Sadock BJ, Samoon A, Sadock VA: Kaplan and Sadock's Pocket Handbook of Clinical Psychiatry, 6th Edition. Philadelphia, PA, Wolters Kluwer, 2019

Salvadore G, Quiroz JA, Machado-Vieira R, et al: The neurobiology of the switch process in bipolar disorder: a review. J Clin Psychiatry 71(11):1488–1501, 2010 20492846

Terao T, Terao M, Yoshimura R, et al: Restless legs syndrome induced by lithium. Biol Psychiatry 30(11):1167–1170, 1991 1777530

Tune LE: Anticholinergic effects of medication in elderly patients. J Clin Psychiatry 62(Suppl 21):11–14, 2001 11584981

Agranulocytosis With Clozapine and Other Psychotropic Medications

Obiora Onwuameze, M.D., Ph.D.
Eric Black, M.D.

Although the literal definition of agranulocytosis is an absence of granulocytes, agranulocytosis is a clinical continuum of neutropenia, or low absolute neutrophil count (ANC). Mild neutropenia is defined as an ANC of 1,000–1,499/µL, and moderate neutropenia is defined as 500–999/µL. Agranulocytosis is a serious emergent clinical state of low ANC with counts of 500/µL or lower. Overall, there are two main types of agranulocytosis, inherited and acquired. Agranulocytosis occurs because of either inadequate production of neutrophils or rapid and abnormal destruction of neutrophils. It is a clinical problem that not only is inherent in the use of psychotropic medications but also can be caused by certain medical conditions and nonpsychotropic medications. In this chapter, we focus on agranulocytosis associated with clozapine and other psychotropic medications.

Psychotropic-induced agranulocytosis is a serious medical problem with an associated fatality rate as high as 7% in some studies (Ibanez et al. 2005). The fatality rate of medication-induced agranulocytosis has decreased in the past 40 years from rates of 20%–50% between 1966 and 2006 (Andersohn et al. 2007). A more recent study reported a fatality rate of 3.1% (Lahdelma and Appelberg 2012). Psychotropic classes associated with agranulocytosis include antipsychotics, antidepressants, mood stabilizers and anticonvulsants, and benzodiazepines (Hoffbrand et al. 1992; Oyesanmi et al. 1999).

In general, the data on the incidence of agranulocytosis for all psychotropics are not available; however, the incidence of all significant hematologic side effects due to psychotropics has been reported to be 1–2 cases per 100,000 patients (Oye-sanmi et al. 1999). The 1-year incidence of agranulocytosis with clozapine ranges from 0.65% to 0.80%, and the incidence is 0.91% for 1.5 years of treatment (Alvir et al. 1993; Ingimarsson et al. 2016; Myles et al. 2018). Data on the epidemiology of psychotropic-induced agranulocytosis indicate that after clozapine, carbamazepine, chlorpromazine, and olanzapine have the highest incidence of agranulocytosis, respectively (Alageel and Gaffas 2016; Fabrazzo et al. 2017). Several factors increase the risk for agranulocytosis, including older age, female sex, genetic susceptibilities, immune dysfunction, impaired renal excretion, severe chronic comorbid medical disorders, and concomitant administration of other psychotropics or medications known to induce agranulocytosis.

Recognition and Detection

Agranulocytosis is a hematologic life-threatening condition that is easily diagnosed by a complete blood count. Failure to appropriately diagnose and intervene can lead to rapid fatality (Hoffbrand et al. 1992). Patients with psychotropic-induced agranulocytosis often present with mouth ulcerations, sore throat, and fever. Patients may also complain of chills, rigors, and chest pain. Vital sign instability can resemble that of patients who are septic.

Culprit Medications

Clozapine and Other Antipsychotics

Agranulocytosis associated with clozapine has been extensively studied. A 2018 meta-analysis of 108 studies reported an incidence rate of 0.9%, which validates previous reports of 0.8% (Myles et al. 2018). The case fatality rate has been reported to be 2.1% (Myles et al. 2018). Although there are no specific data on the incidence rate of agranulocytosis with other atypical antipsychotics, olanzapine, risperidone, quetiapine, and ziprasidone also have been implicated (Flanagan and Dunk 2008). The incidence of agranulocytosis induced by chlorpromazine is estimated to be 0.13% and second only to that of clozapine among antipsychotics. Other typical antipsychotics that have been reported to induce agranulocytosis include haloperidol, fluphenazine, prochlorperazine, promazine, loxapine, and thioridazine (Flanagan and Dunk 2008; Oyesanmi et al. 1999); however, there are no data on the frequency of occurrence.

Antidepressants

Although antidepressant-induced agranulocytosis is rare, with only 10 events reported in the body of literature, several antidepressants have been associated with it. Unfortunately, no data are available on the rate of occurrence for most medications within this class. Among tricyclic antidepressants, nortriptyline, imipramine, clomipramine, and amoxapine have all been reported to induce agranulocytosis (Flanagan and Dunk 2008; Oyesanmi et al. 1999). For monoamine oxidase and serotonin reuptake inhibitors, only tranylcypromine and sertraline have been implicated (Flanagan and Dunk 2008; Oyesanmi et al. 1999; Trescoli-Serrano and Smith 1996). Finally, mirtazapine is the only other antidepressant that has been associated with agranulocytosis, with an incidence rate of 1 per 1,000 patients (Flanagan and Dunk 2008; Oyesanmi et al. 1999).

Mood Stabilizers and Anticonvulsants

Carbamazepine is the mood stabilizer and anticonvulsant with the highest incidence rate of agranulocytosis at 0.5% (Stübner et al. 2004). Several anticonvulsants rarely used in psychiatric care, including ethosuximide, phenytoin, mephenytoin, primidone, and trimethadione, also have been reported to trigger agranulocytosis (Flanagan and Dunk 2008; Oyesanmi et al. 1999). Interestingly, lithium augments granulocyte colony-stimulating factor (G-CSF), increasing the number of granulocytes in agranulocytosis.

Etiology and Pathogenesis

Although the etiopathological mechanism of psychotropic-induced agranulocytosis is not fully understood, the most common mechanism proposed for agranulocytosis associated with clozapine and other psychotropics is suppression of granulopoiesis through the modulation of G-CSF (Malhotra et al. 2015). Supporting this hypothesis, G-CSF is low or undetectable in the plasma of patients presenting with psychotropic-induced agranulocytosis (Flanagan and Dunk 2008; Kendra et al. 1993; Malhotra et al. 2015). Patients with psychotropic-induced agranulocytosis are known to respond quickly to intravenous infusion of G-CSF (Kendra et al. 1993). Given that suppression of granulopoiesis is gradual, most cases of neutropenia and agranulocytosis occur within the first 3–6 months of treatment, although some cases have been reported after 1 week (Andersohn et al. 2007).

Assessment

The clinical setting for initial assessment is dependent on the severity of illness at the time of presentation and may range from an outpatient clinic to an acute or urgent care clinic to the emergency department. On occasion, patients who are hospitalized for other indications may need to be assessed for psychotropic-induced agranulocytosis.

The initial evaluation of agranulocytosis should begin with a thorough current and past medical history and a review of all medications. The capacity of patients to provide a reliable history will depend on the severity of presentation and complications. For those patients who present with altered mental status, collateral information from a reliable informant is necessary.

The presentation of agranulocytosis may be sudden with abrupt onset or may progress gradually. Although some cases of psychotropic-induced agranulocytosis are inadvertently identified during laboratory screening and without clinical symptomatology, patients typically present with signs and symptoms of infection. Symptoms typically include fever and chills, weakness and fatigue, gum inflammation or bleeding, and mouth ulcers. Pharyngitis, with difficulty swallowing, also can occur. The physical examination may show fever greater than 40°C, tachycardia, tachypnea, and hypotension (Mijovic and MacCabe 2020; Sedhai et al. 2021). Patients with an associated respiratory infection may show signs of it on auscultation of the lungs. Findings on the mental state examination vary depending on the severity of complications. Whereas patients with mild symptoms may perform well cognitively, those with more severe disease can have an altered sensorium, psychosis, and agitation.

A complete blood count (CBC) with differential is diagnostic and therefore essential in the initial workup. On a Wright-stained peripheral smear, a decrease or an absence of neutrophils will be apparent. In patients with a relevant history, an erythrocyte sedimentation rate, C-reactive protein test, coagulation studies (prothrombin time, partial thromboplastin time, D-dimer), lactate dehydrogenase test, antinuclear antibody test, rheumatoid factor test, liver function tests, renal function tests, and urine analysis are warranted. If the patient is febrile, cultures of the blood, urine, sputum, and other suspected sites of infection are necessary. Depending on the presentation, a chest X-ray can be considered. After the initial workup, bone marrow aspiration and biopsy can be completed (Sedhai et al. 2021).

Management

Regardless of symptom presentation, when agranulocytosis is confirmed, hospitalization under neutropenic precautions is necessary. A comprehensive multidisciplinary collaborative approach should be the goal, with psychiatry, infectious disease, general internal medicine, and hematology involved in the treatment process. The management plan can be grouped into the following categories with a preventive protocol following clinical stabilization:

1. *Immediate discontinuation of the suspected offending medications.* Once this occurs, agranulocytosis typically resolves within 1–3 weeks.
2. *Use of hematopoietic growth factors.* These medications are used to accelerate the production, maturation, and migration of neutrophils (Andrès et al. 2010). Filgrastim, a G-CSF; sargramostim, a granulocyte-macrophage CSF; and pegfilgrastim, a long-acting filgrastim, are all used to treat agranulocytosis (Lally et al. 2017). As mentioned in the "Mood Stabilizers and Anticonvulsants" subsection, lithium stimulates G-CSF and has been shown to be beneficial for carbamazepine-induced agranulocytosis (Focosi et al. 2009; Oyesanmi et al. 1999).
3. *Management of infection due to agranulocytosis.* In cases of infection, consultation with infectious disease specialists may be warranted (Arnold et al. 2009).

Follow-Up Management

Patients must be monitored with regular repeat CBC with differential. For patients taking clozapine, a required monitored protocol is available through the U.S. FDA Clozapine Risk Evaluation and Mitigation Strategy program: Clozapine_REMS_A_Guide_for_Healthcare_Providers.pdf can be readily accessed via www.clozapinerems.com. In general, for both moderate and severe neutropenia, the CBC with differential should be done daily until the ANC is 1,000/μL or higher and then three times a week until the ANC is 1,500/μL or higher. ANC also should be monitored for 2 weeks after medication discontinuation if the patient's temperature exceeds 38.5°C. For other psychotropic medications, we recommend monthly monitoring for a minimum of 2–3 months, followed by every 3–4 months depending on each patient's specific risks.

Conclusion

Agranulocytosis is a potentially fatal side effect of several psychotropic medications, with the greatest risk being associated with clozapine. Although psychotropic-induced agranulocytosis is rare, patients who are initiated or continued on such medications should be provided with informed consent regarding the risk. Psychoeducation should include a discussion of clinical symptoms associated with agranulocytosis and the need for immediate evaluation if they occur. Patients who are older and female and those with impaired immune states or who are taking concomitant medications that induce agranulocytosis should be made aware of their increased risk.

Key Points

Of all psychiatric medications, clozapine has the highest potential for psychotropic-induced agranulocytosis.

A complete blood count with differential is essential in the diagnosis of agranulocytosis.

Agranulocytosis can be fatal if it is not treated expediently.

The risk of agranulocytosis increases with older age, female sex, use of concomitant medications with a potential for agranulocytosis, and autoimmune or impaired immune states.

The offending agent should be discontinued when the diagnosis of agranulocytosis is expected.

Absolute neutrophil count should be monitored for a specified period after the offending agent is discontinued.

The FDA requires patients who are prescribed clozapine to be monitored in the Clozapine Risk Evaluation and Mitigation Strategy program.

References

Alageel A, Gaffas E: Olanzapine induced neutropenia: rechallenging with olanzapine combined with lithium. Imam Journal of Applied Sciences 1(2):94–99, 2016

Alvir J, Lieberman J, Safferman A, et al: Clozapine-induced agranulocytosis—incidence and risk factors in the United States. N Engl J Med 329:162–167, 1993

Andersohn F, Konzen C, Garbe E: Systematic review: agranulocytosis induced by nonchemotherapy drugs. Ann Intern Med 146(9):657–665, 2007 17470834

Andrès E, Maloisel F, Zimmer J: The role of haematopoietic growth factors granulocyte colony-stimulating factor and granulocyte-macrophage colony-stimulating factor in the management of drug-induced agranulocytosis. Br J Haematol 150(1):3–8, 2010 20151980

Arnold HM, McKinnon PS, Augustin KM, et al: Assessment of an alternative meropenem dosing strategy compared with imipenem-cilastatin or traditional meropenem dosing after cefepime failure or intolerance in adults with neutropenic fever. Pharmacotherapy 29(8):914–923, 2009 19637944

Fabrazzo M, Prisco V, Sampogna G, et al: Clozapine versus other antipsychotics during the first 18 weeks of treatment: a retrospective study on risk factor increase of blood dyscrasias. Psychiatry Res 256:275–282, 2017 28651220

Flanagan RJ, Dunk L: Haematological toxicity of drugs used in psychiatry. Hum Psychopharmacol 23(Suppl 1):27–41, 2008 18098216

Focosi D, Azzarà A, Kast RE, et al: Lithium and hematology: established and proposed uses. J Leukoc Biol 85(1):20–28, 2009 18809733

Hoffbrand AV, Veys PA, Wilkes S: Investigation of psychotropic drug-induced blood agranulocytosis. J Psychopharmacol 6(2):222–224, 1992 22291354

Ibanez L, Vidal X, Ballarin E, Laporte J: Population-based drug-induced agranulocytosis. Arch Intern Med 165:869–874, 2005

Ingimarsson O, Maccabe JH, Haraldsson M, et al: Neutropenia and agranulocytosis during treatment of schizophrenia with clozapine versus other antipsychotics: an observational study in Iceland. BMC Psychiatry 16:441, 2016

Kendra JR, Rugman FP, Flaherty TA, et al: First use of G-CSF in chlorpromazine-induced agranulocytosis: a report of two cases. Postgrad Med J 69(817):885–887, 1993 7507240

Lahdelma L, Appelberg B: Clozapine-induced agranulocytosis in Finland, 1982–2007: long-term monitoring of patients is still warranted. J Clin Psychiatry 73(6):837–842, 2012

Lally J, Malik S, Whiskey E, et al: Clozapine-associated agranulocytosis treatment with granulocyte colony-stimulating factor/ granulocyte-macrophage colony-stimulating factor: a systematic review. J Clin Psychopharmacol 37(4):441–446, 2017 28437295

Malhotra K, Vu P, Wang DH, et al: Olanzapine-induced neutropenia. Ment Illn 7(1):5871, 2015 26266027

Mijovic A, MacCabe JH: Clozapine-induced agranulocytosis. Ann Hematol 99(11):2477–2482, 2020 32815018

Myles N, Myles H, Xia S, et al: Meta-analysis examining the epidemiology of clozapine-associated neutropenia. Acta Psychiatr Scand 138(2):101–109, 2018 29786829

Oyesanmi O, Kunkel EJ, Monti DA, Field HL: Hematologic side effects of psychotropics. Psychosomatics 40(5):414–421, 1999 10479946

Sedhai YR, Lamichhane A, Gupta V: Agranulocytosis. StatPearls, February 6, 2021. Available at: https:// pubmed.ncbi.nlm.nih.gov/32644701. Accessed January 4, 2021.

Stübner S, Grohmann R, Engel R, et al: Blood dyscrasias induced by psychotropic drugs. Pharmacopsychiatry 37(Suppl 1):S70–S78, 2004 15052517

Trescoli-Serrano C, Smith NK: Sertraline-induced agranulocytosis. Postgrad Med J 72(849):446, 1996 8935613

Chapter 4

Benzodiazepines in Combination With Opioids: Therapeutic Benefit Versus Fatal Overdose

Edward Silberman, M.D.

All treatment should be individualized.
—Milton Erickson

Benzodiazepines taken alone are among the safest psychotropic medications, with median lethal dose estimates in the range of several thousand milligrams per kilogram. However, benzodiazepines taken together with opioid medications can be lethal. Benzodiazepines in combination with opioids produce respiratory depression greater than that of either type of medication taken alone, substantially increasing the risk of overdose fatality (Jones et al. 2013). It has been estimated that 60% of drug overdoses occur with prescribed rather than illicitly obtained drugs, that 74% of such overdoses are accidental, and that 75% involve opioids; 29% stem from combined opioid-benzodiazepine use. In one study of chronic pain patients, 85% of those with fatal overdoses had been coprescribed an opioid and a benzodiazepine (Gomes et al. 2011).

Coprescription of opioids and benzodiazepines has been rising in the past few decades. In a national study of ambulatory medical care, the rate at which prescription of both drugs was noted in a single visit quadrupled from 0.5% in 2003 to 2% in 2015 (Agarwal and Landon 2019). Across nine states, 22% of patients who were prescribed an opioid were also prescribed a benzodiazepine at some point, 55% of whom were prescribed both drugs concurrently. More than half of such prescriptions were written by two distinct providers. In parallel, the national rate of overdose from combined opioids and benzodiazepines tripled, from 0.6 deaths per 100,000 in 2004 to 1.7 deaths per 100,000 in 2011 (Guy et al. 2019).

Pain, the essential indication for opioids, and anxiety, the primary indication for benzodiazepines, are well known to occur together frequently and to interact. Patients with chronic pain are twice as likely as those without pain to have an anxiety disorder, especially panic disorder and PTSD; those with multiple pain conditions are especially likely to have comorbid anxiety (Gureje 2008; McWilliams et al. 2003). In addition, anxiety has been associated with decreased pain threshold and pain tolerance, and the presence of either condition may make it more difficult to treat the other (Feeney 2004; Gerrits et al. 2012). Increasing coprescription in the face of risk may therefore reflect the challenges faced by clinicians in treating persistent comorbid conditions.

Recognition and Detection

Any current or recent simultaneous prescription of opioids and benzodiazepines should alert treating clinicians to a potential risk of toxicity or death. Specific clinical profiles are typical of dually prescribed patients. Extreme pain, poor general health, and disability in daily activities have been associated with coprescription of opioids and benzodiazepines (Vadiei and Bhattacharjee 2020). Veterans receiving high-dose benzodiazepines are more likely than those receiving moderate doses to have PTSD, anxiety disorders, and a substance abuse history and to be prescribed concurrent opioid medications (Hermos et al. 2005). Women, middle-aged adults, and those on public insurance may be more likely than others to receive combined treatment, but nonwhite patients may be less likely to do so (Agarwal and Landon 2019). When opioids are concurrently prescribed with benzodiazepines, the total number of days of opioid prescribing and the mean daily dose of opioids tend to be higher when the two medications are prescribed by separate clinicians than when they are prescribed by the same person.

Clinicians should be alert to the possibility that patients may combine a prescription for one type of medication with illegally obtained medication of the other type. In one study, 52% of patients showing evidence of combined use had obtained only one of the drugs through a doctor's prescription (McClure et al. 2017). Of patients in a methadone maintenance program, 25% reported self-initiating benzodiazepines out of curiosity, to relax, to relieve tension or anxiety, to feel good, or to get high (Chen et al. 2011). The risk of death in concurrent users has been found to increase as the daily dose of benzodiazepines increases (Park et al. 2015).

Culprit Medications

Common prescription opioids include morphine, codeine, oxycodone, hydromorphone, fentanyl, hydrocodone, methadone, acetylsalicylic acid+oxycodone, and acetaminophen +hydrocodone. When combined with opioids, both benzodiazepine anxiolytics and Z-drug hypnotics confer increased risk (Szmulewicz et al. 2021; Xu et al. 2021). These include diazepam, chlordiazepoxide, flurazepam, lorazepam, clonazepam, alprazolam, zolpidem, zaleplon, and zopiclone.

Assessment

The Centers for Disease Control and Prevention (CDC) "Guideline for Prescribing Opioids for Chronic Pain" includes the recommendation that "clinicians should avoid prescribing opioid pain medication and benzodiazepines concurrently whenever possible" (Dowell et al. 2016, p. 16). However, the contraindication is not absolute, and coprescription might be appropriate in certain situations, "e.g., severe acute pain in a patient taking long-term, stable low-dose benzodiazepine therapy" (p. 32). Gourlay et al. (2005, p. 109) observed that "in some cases the concurrent use of opioids and sedatives may be quite appropriate while in other cases, this is clearly problematic." They suggested judging on the basis of whether the regimen is improving or worsening the patient's functioning and quality of life.

Clinicians beginning treatment with patients on established combined opioid-benzodiazepine regimens should conduct a thorough psychiatric reassessment to gauge the benefits of a combined regimen compared with other treatments and the risk of such a regimen in the case at hand. Assessments should include verification of all diagnoses, medical comorbidities, history of substance abuse, evidence of benefit and adverse effects of all psychotropic medications, and evidence of the patient's ability to collaborate with clinicians, including their honesty and reliability in use of medications. Recommendations to increase, decrease, taper, add, or withdraw medications should be based on a risk-benefit assessment specific to the case rather than on global population statistics. The assessment of benefits should include functional capacity and quality of life as well as symptom reduction.

Management

No algorithms are available for coprescription of opioids and benzodiazepines. The CDC recommends that the clinician use available prescription monitoring systems to ensure that the patient is taking the medications only as prescribed and consider consulting pharmacists or pain specialists when formulating a treatment plan. Because of the greater medical risk of benzodiazepine withdrawal compared with opioid withdrawal, the CDC recommends tapering the latter first. The CDC also suggests that cognitive-behavioral therapy (CBT) may help patients to successfully complete a taper and that both CBT and antidepressants may be effective substitutes for benzodiazepines in controlling anxiety.

Gourlay et al. (2005) proposed triaging patients by level of risk: patients with no addiction history would be suitable for treatment by a primary care provider; those with a past, but not current, history of addiction or a psychiatric disorder might be treated in primary care with specialist consultation; and those with active substance abuse or untreated psychopathology would need to receive treatment in a specialty setting. When several clinicians are involved, communication among them and careful documentation by all are essential. Gudin et al. (2013) endorsed risk stratification at the outset of treatment, as well as education about the risks and the procedures needed to minimize them. They recommended a formal treatment agreement that summarizes these issues, including routine prescription monitoring checks and periodic unscheduled drug and alcohol tests.

In patients who may be actively abusing substances, Gudin et al. (2013) suggested increasing the frequency of visits and using contingency treatment plans, such as requiring a clean drug test before issuing the next prescription. When nonbenzodiazepine alternatives prove inadequate, doses of opioids and benzodiazepines should be kept as low as possible, the patient should be asked to give informed consent, and documentation of treatment should be meticulous.

A summary of management recommendations for patients taking combined opioid-benzodiazepine regimens is as follows:

- Educate the patient about risks of combined treatment, including the danger of possibly fatal respiratory depression; increased risk with abrupt dose escalation or inconsistent use; and risk of unreported drug and/or substance use, including street drugs, medications prescribed by other clinicians, over-the-counter medications, and alcohol. Document these discussions.
- Monitor for adverse effects, especially drowsiness, respiratory distress, decreased mobility, exercise intolerance, cognitive decline, dyscoordination, and decreased function in life activities.
- Monitor for deviations from prescribed treatment with measures, including periodic unscheduled drug testing and use of a prescription monitoring plan. Standard urine toxicology typically includes assays for amphetamines, cocaine, opioids, benzodiazepines, barbiturates, and cannabis. Alcohol use may be assessed by blood alcohol level or a breath test. Although any deviation from what is prescribed is of concern, the presence of nonprescribed sedatives or alcohol and the absence of a prescribed medication, indicating intermittent use or diversion, are associated with especially high risk. These measures should be explained and agreed to by the patient at the outset of treatment. A formal, signed treatment agreement can be used at the discretion of the clinician, but the discussion with the patient and the results of monitoring should always be documented. Monitoring schedules should fit the known history and risk associated with an individual patient. False-negative tests may occur for benzodiazepines such as lorazepam and clonazepam that are not metabolized to oxazepam, which the standard assays detect. When there are discrepancies between laboratory results

and the patient's report, clinical pathology specialists should be consulted about the likelihood of false-positive and false-negative results and the availability of confirmatory tests.

- Take action to mitigate high risk. When patients experience concerning adverse effects of prescribed treatment or inability to cooperate with treatment, the treatment plan should be modified on the basis of the specifics of the case. Increased risk indicators for respiratory depression require lowering the opioid, the benzodiazepine, or both. Which to taper first should be determined by the patient's history of symptoms and therapeutic response. Prescribing naloxone in the form of Narcan, which can easily be self-administered by patients experiencing symptoms of opioid toxicity, may also mitigate the risk. Patients who show an inability to cooperate adequately with treatment, either by taking medications other than as prescribed or by using other substances, may present unacceptable risk for combined opioid-benzodiazepine therapy. When there is pressure of time, it is generally easier to taper opioids quickly, on a fixed schedule, than benzodiazepines; in addition, opioids are the more powerful respiratory depressants.

- Consider substitute therapy. Nonopioid analgesic medications may be effective for chronic noncancer pain, and a wide range of medications, including antidepressants, buspirone, anticonvulsants, β-blockers, and second-generation neuroleptics, may mitigate anxiety. Psychotherapy and behavioral approaches may contribute to treatment of both chronic pain and chronic anxiety. Clinicians should attempt to engage patients in trials of these treatments when dual prescription is no longer feasible.

- Use flexible benzodiazepine tapers. Anxiety patients are concerned about control, as well as having to deal with both withdrawal phenomena and possible return of untreated anxiety. Taper should start with a clear, nonpejorative explanation of its necessity. A plausible initial taper schedule is 25% every 2 weeks, but patients should be assured that there is no hurry and that they will not need to take the next step down until they are comfortable where they are. Patients experience proportional, not absolute, dose changes, so taper steps often need to be reduced as the total daily dose decreases.

- Communicate with coprescribers. When another clinician is prescribing the opioids, set up lines of communication, including an initial discussion and periodic follow-ups. Such communication should be documented.

Patients taking opioids alone may have severe chronic anxiety. Adding a benzodiazepine is not contraindicated absolutely, but such patients should have high need and low behavioral risk; they should have tried a variety of other plausible treatment options without success, be substantially impaired by anxiety symptoms, not be actively abusing substances, and have a record of good cooperation with treatment. It is important to educate patients about what to expect from anxiolytic medications. Except for panic attacks, medications do not eradicate anxiety; they only moderate it and often need to be supplemented by nonmedical therapies. Informed consent for benefits and risks should be documented.

Good responders should not need more than 2–4 mg/day of a high-potency benzodiazepine for optimal treatment, and combined therapy may necessitate keeping the dose lower. People who are equivocal in describing benefits are not likely to be good benzodiazepine responders. A higher dose is unlikely to help and increases risk.

Follow-Up Management

Chronic pain and chronic anxiety are more likely to respond to an incremental approach than to attempts to find a magic bullet. Long-term patients should be educated about the limitations of medications and the need to seek small, stepwise changes in outlook and behavior that will gradually improve their quality of life. Regular follow-up with the prescribing clinician that includes such discussions may be sufficient, but formal procedures, such as CBT, may facilitate the process of gradual change. Prescribers should keep in mind that anticipatory anxiety is an almost universal complication of both pain syndromes and anxiety disorders. As patients stabilize or gradually improve, their fear of being overwhelmed by unbearable symptoms gradually diminishes, possibly lessening their need for medication. Therefore, long-term treatment should include consideration of attempts at gradual, flexible reduction of the dose of either or both medications. Such discussions should be collaborative, and decisions about dose reduction should be mutual and free of pressure or moralizing undertone.

Key Points

Opioid-benzodiazepine regimens convey high risk for toxicity.

Despite the risk, combined regimens may be best for some patients.

Alternatives should be shown to have failed before a patient starts combined treatment.

Risk is lowest with low to moderate, stable doses of both medications.

Doses should be changed slowly.

Risk should be reassessed at each step.

Patients should be monitored for use that deviates from what is prescribed.

Patients found to be unreliable should not be prescribed combined treatment.

References

Agarwal SD, Landon BE: Patterns in outpatient benzodiazepine prescribing in the United States. JAMA Netw Open 2(1):e187399, 2019 30681713

Chen KW, Berger CC, Forde DP, et al: Benzodiazepine use and misuse among patients in a methadone program. BMC Psychiatry 11:90, 2011 21595945

Dowell D, Haegerich T, Chou R: CDC guideline for prescribing opioids for chronic pain—United States, 2016. MMWR Recomm Rep 65(1):1–49, 2016 26987082

Feeney SL: The relationship between pain and negative affect in older adults: anxiety as a predictor of pain. J Anxiety Disord 18(6):733–744, 2004 15474849

Gerrits MMJG, Vogelzangs N, van Oppen P, et al: Impact of pain on the course of depressive and anxiety disorders. Pain 153(2):429–436, 2012 22154919

Gomes T, Mamdani MM, Dhalla IA, et al: Opioid dose and drug-related mortality in patients with nonmalignant pain. Arch Intern Med 171(7):686–691, 2011 21482846

Gourlay DL, Heit HA, Almahrezi A: Universal precautions in pain medicine: a rational approach to the treatment of chronic pain. Pain Med 6(2):107–112, 2005 15773874

Gudin JA, Mogali S, Jones JD, et al: Risks, management, and monitoring of combination opioid, benzodiazepines, and/or alcohol use. Postgrad Med 125(4):115–130, 2013 23933900

Gureje O: Comorbidity of pain and anxiety disorders. Curr Psychiatry Rep 10(4):318–322, 2008 18627670

Guy GP Jr, Zhang K, Halpin J, et al: An examination of concurrent opioid and benzodiazepine prescribing in 9 states, 2015. Am J Prev Med 57(5):629–636, 2019 31564606

Hermos JA, Young MM, Lawler EV, et al: Characterizations of long-term anxiolytic benzodiazepine prescriptions in veteran patients. J Clin Psychopharmacol 25(6):600–604, 2005 16282847

Jones CM, Mack KA, Paulozzi LJ: Pharmaceutical overdose deaths, United States, 2010. JAMA 309(7):657–659, 2013 23423407

McClure FL, Niles JK, Kaufman HW, et al: Concurrent use of opioids and benzodiazepines: evaluation of prescription drug monitoring by a United States laboratory. J Addict Med 11(6):420–426, 2017 28953504

McWilliams LA, Cox BJ, Enns MW: Mood and anxiety disorders associated with chronic pain: an examination in a nationally representative sample. Pain 106(1-2):127–133, 2003 14581119

Park TW, Saitz R, Ganoczy D, et al: Benzodiazepine prescribing patterns and deaths from drug overdose among US veterans receiving opioid analgesics: case-cohort study. BMJ 350:h2698, 2015 26063215

Szmulewicz A, Bateman BT, Levin R, et al: The risk of overdose with concomitant use of Z-drugs and prescription opioids: a population-based cohort study. Am J Psychiatry 178(7):643–650, 2021 33900810

Vadiei N, Bhattacharjee S: Concurrent opioid and benzodiazepine utilization patterns and predictors among community-dwelling adults in the United States. Psychiatr Serv 71(10):1011–1019, 2020 32517642

Xu KY, Borodovsky JT, Presnall N, et al: Association between benzodiazepine or Z-drug prescriptions and drug-related poisonings among patients receiving buprenorphine maintenance: a case-crossover analysis. Am J Psychiatry 178(7):651–659, 2021 33653119

Cardiac Emergencies Such as Arrhythmias, QTc Prolongation, and Cardiomyopathy

Margo C. Funk, M.D., M.A.
Junyang Lou, M.D., Ph.D.

Urgent and emergent adverse cardiac events may occur with the use of certain psychotropic medications. Potentially fatal events include sudden cardiac death from tachyarrhythmias, including ventricular tachycardia and ventricular fibrillation; bradyarrhythmia and asystole from conduction disturbance and heart block; and hypotension and multiorgan failure from ischemia and depressed ventricular function.

Torsades de Pointes

Torsades de pointes (TdP) is a polymorphic ventricular tachycardia that occurs in the setting of prolonged ventricular repolarization and may result in sudden cardiac death, often presaged by prolongation of the QTc interval on the 12-lead electrocardiogram (ECG). Direct, drug-induced blockade of potassium efflux from the cardiac myocyte can result in TdP in the presence of other risk factors, including female sex, older age, bradycardia, hypokalemia, hypomagnesemia, hypocalcemia, renal or hepatic dysfunction, family history of sudden cardiac death, personal history of heart disease or prior TdP, and the coadministration of other QTc-prolonging medications or medications with cytochrome P450 (CYP) inhibition of QTc-prolonging substrates.

Recognition and Detection

Symptoms of TdP include light-headedness, syncope and pre-syncope, seizurelike episodes, and aborted sudden cardiac death. TdP manifests on the ECG as a wide complex tachycardia with a characteristic alternation of QRS amplitude around the isoelectric baseline. TdP often goes undetected unless captured by telemetry or ECG or through interrogation of cardiac implanted electronic devices, such as permanent cardiac pacemakers and implantable cardioverter defibrillators. A common electrocardiographic precursor to TdP is bradycardia with QTc prolongation, abnormal T-wave morphology, and frequent premature ventricular contractions.

Culprit Medications

Methadone is in the highest risk category of all medications known to cause TdP. Other high-risk psychotropic medications include certain antipsychotics, such as low-potency phenothiazines (chlorpromazine, thioridazine, mesoridazine), ziprasidone, and iloperidone.

Despite intravenous haloperidol's reputation, a paucity of data supports the assertion that it confers considerable risk for TdP. There has never been a thorough QT/QTc study of intravenous haloperidol or a head-to-head comparison with the oral formulation, which is considered to have moderate risk of QTc prolongation (Beach et al. 2020).

Citalopram and, to a lesser extent, escitalopram prolong the QTc interval enough to differ from other selective serotonin reuptake inhibitors but confer low risk for TdP. Tricyclic antidepressants (TCAs) also have been historically associated with QTc prolongation, but more recent evidence suggests that this observation may be confounded by tachycardia-related overestimation of QTc in studies of TCA overdose (Noordam et al. 2015).

Assessment

TdP risk can be assessed with continuous telemetry, ECG, or interrogation of cardiac implanted electronic devices. Serum K^+ and Mg^{2+} levels and scrutiny of medication administration records can also be used to check for TdP risk.

Management

Acute management of TdP should be guided by the advanced cardiac life support algorithm, which includes treatment with defibrillation, epinephrine, and intravenous Mg^{2+} and, in some cases, treatment of bradycardia with transcutaneous or transvenous cardiac overdrive pacing or isoproterenol.

Follow-Up Management

In the setting of ongoing QTc prolongation or following an episode of TdP, a careful risk-benefit analysis needs to be performed, weighing the cardiac risks of continuing a potentially high-risk psychotropic medication against the psychiatric morbidity of its discontinuation. Mitigation of modifiable TdP risk factors should be undertaken, including repletion of serum K^+ (goal≥4.0 mEq/L) and serum Mg^{2+} (goal≥2.0 mg/dL), avoidance of additional QTc-prolonging medications, and consultation with cardiac electrophysiology (Funk et al. 2020).

Brugada Syndrome

Brugada syndrome is estimated to account for 20% of sudden cardiac death in patients with structurally normal hearts. The inherited form of the syndrome is often acquired through transmission of an autosomal dominant mutation of the sodium channel gene *SCN5A*, which encodes for the α-subunit of the cardiac sodium channel. The acquired form of the syndrome may occur in the presence of certain medications, primarily sodium channel blockers, which may unmask the characteristic ECG pattern of Brugada syndrome.

Recognition and Detection

Signs and symptoms of Brugada syndrome include syncope, seizure, nocturnal agonal respirations, and aborted sudden cardiac death. Some patients may be asymptomatic. The ECG is characterized by coved ST-segment elevation of 2 mm or greater, followed by a negative T wave (known as type 1 Brugada pattern).

Culprit Medications

Sodium channel blockers include TCAs (specifically amitriptyline, clomipramine, desipramine, nortriptyline), lithium, loxapine, trifluoperazine, oxcarbazepine, lamotrigine, carbamazepine, cocaine, and cannabis (Rastogi et al. 2020).

Assessment

Brugada syndrome can be assessed with ECG and electro-physiological studies.

Management

Immediate placement of an implantable cardioverter defibrillator is warranted in patients presenting with aborted sudden cardiac death and in other symptomatic patients in whom an extracardiac cause is not identified. Asymptomatic patients with a type 1 Brugada pattern on ECG should receive an implantable cardioverter defibrillator if they have a positive family history of sudden cardiac death worrisome for Brugada syndrome and if electrophysiological studies induce ventricular tachycardia (Antzelevitch et al. 2005).

Follow-Up Management

Asymptomatic patients with no family history of sudden cardiac death and an induced type 1 Brugada pattern do not need implantable cardioverter defibrillators but should be closely followed up by cardiology specialists. The offending sodium channel–blocking medication must be discontinued.

Sick Sinus Syndrome (Sinus Node Dysfunction)

Sick sinus syndrome, also known as sinus node dysfunction, may occur in relation to older age, idiopathic degenerative fibrosis, ischemia, inflammatory and infiltrative cardiomyopathy, scarring from cardiac surgery or procedures, neuromuscular conditions, rare genetic conditions, and medication effects typically from calcium channel blockers and β-blockers.

Recognition and Detection

Signs and symptoms of sick sinus syndrome may include fatigue, light-headedness, presyncope and syncope, dyspnea, chest discomfort, altered mental status, palpitations, skipped beats, and lack of heart rate increase with physical activity. An ECG may show sinus bradycardia, sinus arrest, bradycardia-tachycardia syndrome, sinoatrial exit block, and atrial fibrillation with slow ventricular response.

Culprit Medications

Lithium has been associated with sick sinus syndrome (Mehta and Vannozzi 2017).

Assessment

Sick sinus syndrome can be assessed with an ECG, cardiac event monitor, exercise stress test, and serum lithium level.

Management

If medications are suspected to be the cause of sick sinus syndrome, adjusting the dosage or changing to an alternative medication is warranted. Most patients eventually need a permanent cardiac pacemaker.

Follow-Up Management

Patients with sick sinus syndrome should be closely followed up by cardiology specialists.

Atrioventricular Block

Atrioventricular (AV) block is a disturbance of the regular cardiac conduction pathway at the AV node. AV block can be triggered by myocardial ischemia, cardiomyopathy, surgery, and drug toxicity—typically, calcium channel blockers and other AV node–blocking agents. First-degree AV block is not an emergency. Second-degree AV block is characterized by two types: Mobitz type I (Wenckebach) and Mobitz type II. Mobitz type I often occurs in healthy individuals and is typically not an emergency, whereas type II often occurs in patients with known structural heart disease and requires urgent management. Third-degree AV block is an emergency and represents complete dissociation of electrical conduction from the atria to the ventricles.

Recognition and Detection

Signs and symptoms of AV block include fatigue, dyspnea, presyncope and syncope, chest pain, bradycardia, hypotension, diaphoresis, pallor, altered mental status, obtundation, retraction, cool skin, and decreased capillary refill. ECG characterization is as follows:

- Mobitz type I block: gradual prolongation of the PR interval over a few cardiac cycles until an atrial impulse is blocked, manifesting as a P wave without a subsequent QRS complex
- Mobitz type II block: constant PR intervals with intermittent blockade of atrial impulses
- Third-degree AV block: complete dissociation of atrial and ventricular impulses with independent atrial and ventricular (escape) rates

Culprit Medications

Culprit medications include calcium channel blockers (TCAs, benzodiazepines, lithium, clozapine, carbamazepine, citalopram) (Arroyo Plasencia et al. 2012; Zahradník et al. 2008) and CYP2D6 inhibitors such as paroxetine, fluoxetine, and bupropion in combination with some β-blockers (metoprolol, carvedilol, nebivolol, propranolol).

Assessment

AV block can be assessed with ECG, telemetry, serum electrolytes, complete blood count, and digoxin level, if indicated. If ischemia is suspected, cardiac biomarkers (troponin, creatine kinase–myocardial bound) should be measured. Electrophysiological testing may be warranted.

Management

Patients with second- and third-degree blocks require hospitalization and monitoring. For Mobitz type I, treatment is not usually required; however, bradycardia and hypotension typically respond to atropine (0.5 mg IV, may be repeated) or may require transcutaneous or transvenous pacing. Mobitz type II and third-degree block require pacing immediately after the rhythm is identified and until a permanent cardiac pacemaker can be placed. Bradycardia and hypotension with third-degree block may not respond to atropine and may instead require dopamine and epinephrine. Offending medications should be discontinued.

Follow-Up Management

First-degree AV block and second-degree Mobitz type I require a permanent cardiac pacemaker only if the patient is symptomatic. Second-degree Mobitz type II nearly always requires a permanent cardiac pacemaker, and third-degree block always requires one.

Ventricular Conduction Delay

Ventricular conduction delay refers to impaired electrical conduction through the His-Purkinje system that is often due to sodium channel blockade, resulting in slowed, cell-to-cell depolarization of the myocardium. A widened QRS complex at 110 ms or greater is suggestive of sodium channel blockade and is a predictor of life-threatening cardiac events, including bradyarrhythmia, complete heart block (i.e., AV block), ventricular tachycardia, and ventricular fibrillation (Agrawal et al. 2008).

Recognition and Detection

Ventricular conduction delay is recognized by widening of the QRS complex (QRS≥110 ms) on ECG, including interventricular conduction delay (QRS=110–119 ms) and bundle branch block (QRS≥120 ms).

Culprit Medications

Culprit medications include sodium channel blockers, especially in overdose (TCAs, lamotrigine, carbamazepine, cocaine).

Assessment

Ventricular conduction delay can be assessed with ECG.

Management

Offending medications should be discontinued.

Follow-Up Management

Patients should avoid future use of sodium channel–blocking medications.

Myocarditis

Myocarditis is an inflammatory disorder of the myocardium that causes myocyte damage or degeneration. Medication-induced myocarditis is typically an eosinophilic hypersensitivity reaction.

Recognition and Detection

Signs and symptoms of myocarditis include low to moderate fever, dyspnea, palpitations, tachycardia, flulike illness, nausea, dizziness, and, occasionally, chest pain.

Culprit Medications

Clozapine is the most common culprit medication. Rare cases of myocarditis with olanzapine, lamotrigine, and TCAs have been reported.

Assessment

Myocarditis can be assessed with ECG, cardiac biomarkers (troponin, creatine kinase–myocardial bound), C-reactive protein, white blood cell count, and imaging including echocardiography and cardiac MRI. Endomyocardial biopsy is the gold standard for diagnosis; however, its use is limited because of the invasive nature of the procedure and risk of complications.

Management

Acute management involves hemodynamic support and preservation of cardiac function. Medication management includes diuretics, β-blockers, angiotensin converting enzyme inhibitors, and corticosteroids.

Follow-Up Management

Prophylactic baseline ECG prior to clozapine initiation followed by weekly ECG, troponin, C-reactive protein, and vital sign screening for the first 4 weeks of treatment may be helpful for early detection. Clozapine rechallenge after myocarditis is poorly studied, with only a few successful case reports in patients with recovered left ventricular ejection fraction of 50% or more. Rechallenge should be attempted on only a case-by-case basis in collaboration with cardiology with slow dose titration by 25 mg weekly, twice-weekly monitoring of cardiac biomarkers for 8 weeks, and transthoracic echocardiography every 6 months (Griffin et al. 2021).

Noninflammatory Cardiomyopathy

Cardiomyopathy is a disorder of dysfunctional myocardial contractility that results in a reduced left-ventricular ejection fraction.

Recognition and Detection

Signs and symptoms of cardiomyopathy include dyspnea, chest pain, palpitations, tachycardia, and fatigue.

Culprit Medications

Clozapine is the most common culprit medication. Rare cases have been reported with lithium.

Assessment

Cardiomyopathy can be assessed with echocardiography and B-type natriuretic peptide.

Management

Acute management is supportive to minimize the risk of heart failure and to optimize cardiac function. Medication management includes use of diuretics, β-blockers, angiotensin converting enzyme inhibitors, and corticosteroids.

Follow-Up Management

Clozapine rechallenge is not typically recommended in the setting of critical left-ventricular dysfunction.

Coronary Vasospasm

Coronary vasospasm is a type of chest pain syndrome that may occur with use of certain medications that increase activity of the sympathetic nervous system.

Recognition and Detection

Signs and symptoms of coronary vasospasm include chest discomfort, pressure, and/or pain in the substernal or epigastric areas that often occur at rest and often radiate to the neck, jaw, left shoulder, or left arm. Women and elderly individuals may present with dyspnea, nausea, vomiting, diaphoresis, and unexplained fatigue.

Culprit Medications

Culprit medications include prescribed (amphetamine, dextroamphetamine, methylphenidate, dexmethylphenidate, lisdexamfetamine) and illicit (e.g., methamphetamine, cocaine) stimulants and cannabis.

Assessment

Coronary vasospasm can be assessed with serial ECGs and cardiac biomarkers (troponin, creatine kinase–myocardial bound, myoglobin).

Management

Acute treatment includes supplemental oxygen, nitroglycerin, and morphine sulfate. Patients with persistent ST elevation should be evaluated for immediate reperfusion therapy. Vasodilators (calcium channel blockers, long-acting nitroglycerin) are used to treat coronary vasospasm. Offending medication should be discontinued.

Follow-Up Management

Follow-up management should include lifestyle modification; smoking cessation, if applicable; and cardiology follow-up.

Conclusion

Psychiatrists should be aware of potentially life-threatening cardiac adverse events from the use of certain psychotropic medications. Psychiatrists should be able to recognize signs and symptoms of these entities, identify basic electrocardiographic abnormalities such as QTc prolongation and widening of the QRS complex, and perform collaborative psychiatric treatment planning following a cardiac emergency.

Key Points

Psychiatrists should be aware of potentially life-threatening cardiac adverse events from the use of psychotropic medications.

Psychiatrists should be able to identify basic electrocardiographic abnormalities such as QTc prolongation and widening of the QRS complex.

Psychiatry and cardiology collaboration is essential following a cardiac emergency in patients taking psychotropic medications.

References

Agrawal P, Nadel ES, Brown DFM: Tricyclic antidepressant overdose. J Emerg Med 34(3):321–325, 2008 18296006

Antzelevitch C, Brugada P, Borggrefe M, et al: Brugada syndrome: report of the second consensus conference. Heart Rhythm 2(4):429–440, 2005 15898165

Arroyo Plasencia AM, Ballentine LM, Mowry JB, Kao LW: Benzodiazepine-associated atrioventricular block. Am J Ther 19(1):e48–e52, 2012 20535011

Beach SR, Gross AF, Hartney KE, et al: Intravenous haloperidol: a systematic review of side effects and recommendations for clinical use. Gen Hosp Psychiatry 67:42–50, 2020 32979582

Funk MC, Beach SR, Bostwick JR, et al: QTc prolongation and psychotropic medications. Am J Psychiatry 177(3):273–274, 2020 32114782

Griffin JM, Woznica E, Gilotra NA, et al: Clozapine-associated myocarditis: a protocol for monitoring upon clozapine initiation and recommendations for how to conduct a clozapine rechallenge. J Clin Psychopharmacol 41(2):180–185, 2021 33587399

Mehta N, Vannozzi R: Lithium-induced electrocardiographic changes: a complete review. Clin Cardiol 40(12):1363–1367, 2017 29247520

Noordam R, van den Berg ME, Niemeijer MN, et al: Assessing prolongation of the heart rate corrected QT interval in users of tricyclic antidepressants: advice to use Fridericia rather than Bazett's correction. J Clin Psychopharmacol 35(3):260–265, 2015 25856783

Rastogi A, Viani-Walsh D, Akbari S, et al: Pathogenesis and management of Brugada syndrome in schizophrenia: a scoping review. Gen Hosp Psychiatry 67:83–91, 2020 33065406

Zahradník I, Minarovič I, Zahradníková A: Inhibition of the cardiac L-type calcium channel current by antidepressant drugs. J Pharmacol Exp Ther 324(3):977–984, 2008 18048694

Discontinuation of Psychotropic Medications

Vladan Starcevic, M.D., Ph.D., FRANZCP

Discontinuing a psychotropic medication is common in clinical practice. It occurs for several reasons, including adverse effects of the drug, the patient's decision to stop the medication, and planned cessation (because of, e.g., a lack of effectiveness, a change to another pharmacological agent, sustained remission, or pregnancy).

Decreasing the dose of a medication or its discontinuation can be accompanied by three types of symptoms (Chouinard and Chouinard 2015). The first type of symptoms are referred to as *rebound symptoms,* which denote reappearance of the symptoms for which the medication was prescribed, usually with a greater intensity than before the onset of treatment. Rebound symptoms occur within days of the change in the medication regimen and typically disappear within 6 weeks. The second type of symptoms relate to the emergence of new symptoms, that is, those that were not present before commencing pharmacological treatment and before decreasing the dose or ceasing the medication. These are characterized as *withdrawal symptoms* and usually have an onset, duration, and outcome similar to those of rebound symptoms. The third type of symptoms are those encompassed by the term *persistent postwithdrawal disorder*; this represents any combination of rebound and withdrawal symptoms that occur up to 6 weeks after the change in the medication regimen and persist for prolonged periods of time (often for more than 6 weeks) and are potentially irreversible.

In addition to these consequences of medication discontinuation, once the medication has been stopped, there is a risk of relapse of the condition for which the medication was originally prescribed. Relapse can occur *at any time* after medication cessation, and it is important to keep this in mind when distinguishing between various withdrawal and rebound symptoms, on the one hand, and symptoms of relapse, on the other.

In this chapter, I address changes that occur in the context of discontinuation of various types of psychotropic medications: antipsychotics, mood stabilizers, antidepressants, and benzodiazepines and nonbenzodiazepine hypnotics (Z-drugs).

Discontinuation of Antipsychotic Medications

Recognition and Detection

Withdrawal Symptoms

A wide variety of withdrawal symptoms have been described following the discontinuation of both first-generation antipsychotics (FGAs) and second-generation antipsychotics (SGAs), with a frequency of approximately 23% (Cerovecki et al. 2013). The nature of these symptoms depends on the pharmacodynamic characteristics of the specific medication; the course is favorable, with complete recovery usually occurring within days or several weeks.

Rebound Symptoms

Worsening of psychotic symptoms immediately after discontinuation of both FGAs and SGAs has been reported in 36% of patients (Cerovecki et al. 2013). Rebound symptoms may be more common after rapid cessation of clozapine and quetiapine.

Persistent Postwithdrawal Disorder

There are two types of persistent postwithdrawal disorder: tardive dyskinesia and supersensitivity psychosis (Chouinard and Chouinard 2008). The former is characterized by various involuntary, repetitive, and purposeless movements (e.g., orofacial dyskinesia and choreiform movements) and has been associated mainly with the use of FGAs. By contrast, supersensitivity psychosis has been reported following the cessation of both FGAs and SGAs; its features vary from one patient to another, and they are often accompanied by abnormal involuntary movements.

Assessment

Symptoms are assessed through patient reporting or active questioning, physical examination if necessary, and Abnormal Involuntary Movement Scale (AIMS) testing for tardive dyskinesia.

Management

Antipsychotic medications should be discontinued gradually (over a period of several weeks to several months) to prevent withdrawal and rebound symptoms and decrease the risk of relapse. However, this approach is not always successful, and it is not effective for the prevention of tardive dyskinesia and supersensitivity psychosis. Rebound psychotic symptoms may need to be treated with the same or a different antipsychotic agent, depending on the duration and severity of such symptoms. Tardive dyskinesia has been notoriously difficult to treat, but the vesicular monoamine transporter type 2 (VMAT2) inhibitors valbenazine (40 or 80 mg/day) and deutetrabenazine (24–48 mg/day) have improved outcomes and are approved for treatment of tardive dyskinesia. Supersensitivity psychosis is usually resistant to the originally used antipsychotic medication and may respond to another antipsychotic, possibly in combination with an anticonvulsant.

Follow-Up Management

Persistent tardive dyskinesia and supersensitivity psychosis often require a flexible management approach and adjustments in the type of pharmacological agents used and their doses. After discontinuation of antipsychotic medications, patients are at higher risk for relapse of their psychotic illness, which calls for ongoing supportive measures, psychosocial interventions, and careful follow-up.

Discontinuation of Mood Stabilizers

Lithium

Recognition and Detection

Although uncommon, withdrawal symptoms of lithium include tremor, polyuria, polydipsia, muscular weakness, and dry mouth. These are similar to the adverse effects of lithium, so establishing the cause is crucial. Psychiatric symptoms associated with discontinuation may include anxiety, nervousness, irritability, elevated mood, mania, and depressed mood, accompanied by sleep difficulties.

Assessment

Symptoms are assessed through patient reporting or active questioning.

Management

To prevent withdrawal symptoms and decrease the risk for relapse, lithium should be tapered very slowly, preferably over several months. If this is not possible (e.g., when adverse effects of lithium are prominent), the use of another mood stabilizer may be considered. Withdrawal symptoms usually do not require specific treatment because they typically diminish in intensity and disappear within several days.

Follow-Up Management

The risk of relapse of bipolar disorder after lithium discontinuation is high, especially if lithium has been ceased quickly (within 2 weeks). Therefore, patients need to be closely monitored for any symptoms and signs of relapse after lithium discontinuation.

Anticonvulsants

Recognition and Detection

Data are limited on withdrawal symptoms after cessation of anticonvulsants (valproate, carbamazepine, lamotrigine) used as mood stabilizers. Overall, these symptoms appear to be uncommon, nonspecific, and mild. However, abrupt withdrawal of anticonvulsants may be accompanied by seizures, especially in patients with epilepsy or a history of seizures.

Assessment

Symptoms are assessed through patient reporting or active questioning and observation of any seizure activity.

Management

Gradual cessation (over several weeks to a few months) is recommended mainly to decrease the risk of relapse of bipolar disorder.

Follow-Up Management

Given the high risk for relapse of bipolar disorder after discontinuation of all mood stabilizers, a careful follow-up of patients who ceased anticonvulsants as mood stabilizers is necessary.

Discontinuation of Antidepressants

Withdrawal symptoms have been reported after tapering and cessation of all classes of antidepressant medications, with a frequency ranging from 27% to 86%, with a weighted average of 56% (Davies and Read 2019). Withdrawal symptoms following the discontinuation of tricyclic antidepressants and irreversible monoamine oxidase inhibitors have been well described, which has led to a recommendation to taper these agents before their cessation. Given the much lower frequency with which these agents have been used in recent decades, most of the attention in the realm of antidepressant discontinuation has focused on selective serotonin reuptake inhibitors (SSRIs) and serotonin-norepinephrine reuptake inhibitors (SNRIs). Symptoms that have been reported following the discontinuation of other antidepressants (i.e., mirtazapine, mianserin, trazodone, agomelatine, bupropion, vilazodone, vortioxetine) do not seem to be common or to have clinical significance. Nevertheless, a gradual reduction in the dose of these agents before their cessation is probably prudent.

Recognition and Detection of Discontinuation Difficulties With SSRIs and SNRIs

Withdrawal Symptoms

After discontinuation of SSRIs and SNRIs, the relatively specific withdrawal manifestations include unusual sensory experiences, such as electrical shock–like sensations (often described as *brain zaps*) and visual trails or prolonged afterimages (palinopsia); dizziness; imbalance; various difficulties with coordination; and genital hypersensitivity. Other withdrawal symptoms, although common, are generally much less specific and include flulike symptoms (e.g., headache, chills, sweating, weakness, lethargy, fatigue), insomnia, nausea, vomiting, stomach cramps, diarrhea, numbness or tingling sensations, dysesthesias, muscle cramps or pains, and unsteady gait. Withdrawal symptoms are more common and more severe after stopping paroxetine (because of its shorter elimination half-life) and venlafaxine and least common after fluoxetine cessation (because of its longer elimination half-life).

Rebound Symptoms

Rebound depressive and anxiety symptoms have been observed after discontinuation of SSRIs and SNRIs, with these symptoms being more likely following paroxetine and venlafaxine cessation than after fluoxetine cessation.

Persistent Postwithdrawal Disorder

Although persistent postwithdrawal symptoms do not appear to be common, they can be severe, and their outcome may be uncertain. The most frequent features include various mood and somatic symptoms, followed by sleep disturbance and cognitive difficulties (Hengartner et al. 2020). Some reports suggest that these symptoms may occur more often after cessation of paroxetine and venlafaxine, but other research indicates that the risk is not associated with any particular SSRI or SNRI (Hengartner et al. 2020).

Assessment of Discontinuation Difficulties With SSRIs and SNRIs

Symptoms are assessed through patient reporting or active questioning and physical examination if necessary.

Management of Discontinuation Difficulties With SSRIs and SNRIs

The usual approach to discontinuation of SSRIs and SNRIs has been a slow and individualized tapering to decrease the risk of withdrawal and rebound symptoms. The initial process of tapering is usually better tolerated than discontinuing the medication. If the withdrawal symptoms occur during taper, the discontinuation process may be paused temporarily, or the dose may need to be increased, with taper then attempted at a slower rate. Paroxetine should be tapered more slowly than fluoxetine, but there are major differences between patients in terms of the rate at which doses of SSRIs and SNRIs can be safely decreased. The practice of replacing paroxetine or another SSRI with fluoxetine before the cessation of SSRIs is not supported by evidence (e.g., Fava and Belaise 2018).

It has been suggested that hyperbolic tapering based on serotonin transporter occupancy might greatly reduce the risk of withdrawal symptoms (Horowitz and Taylor 2019), especially in patients who previously had great difficulties with tapering or ceasing antidepressants. This method consists of progressively smaller reductions in doses as the total daily dosage decreases, possibly with longer intervals between reduction steps. However, the method has not been tested, and it may be difficult to implement it in routine clinical practice because of the extremely low doses (e.g., 0.37 mg of citalopram) that need to be administered just before completely ceasing the medication. It is unclear how to manage persistent postwithdrawal symptoms other than attempting to alleviate the specific symptoms.

Follow-Up Management of Discontinuation Difficulties With SSRIs and SNRIs

Patients who stopped taking SSRIs or SNRIs may be more likely to relapse than those who continue taking them. Monitoring for the manifestations of relapse is important, as is distinguishing between true relapse and various features of persistent postwithdrawal disorder. A relapse of major depressive or anxiety disorder may or may not respond to the same SSRI or SNRI.

Discontinuation of Benzodiazepines and Z-Drugs

Although there are more data on benzodiazepine discontinuation than on the cessation of Z-drugs (zolpidem, zopiclone, eszopiclone, zaleplon), it seems that in this regard these agents are more alike than different (Cosci and Chouinard 2020).

Recognition and Detection

Withdrawal Symptoms

After discontinuation of benzodiazepines, the relatively specific withdrawal symptoms include hypersensitivity to light, sound, smell, or taste; an unpleasant feeling of movement as if being on a boat or walking on waves; ringing in the ears; distorted body image; various other perceptual disturbances; and dissociative symptoms. If present, these symptoms may be useful for identification of benzodiazepine withdrawal. Although rare, seizures are the most serious withdrawal symptom. Other withdrawal symptoms include nausea, vomiting and other gastrointestinal distress, flulike symptoms, sweating, weakness, tachycardia, tremor, muscle pain, confusion, restlessness, insomnia, and even psychotic symptoms (i.e., hallucinations, paranoia). Withdrawal symptoms are more common and more severe after an abrupt discontinuation of high-potency benzodiazepines with a short to medium elimination half-life (i.e., alprazolam, lorazepam, oxazepam, bromazepam).

Rebound Symptoms

Rebound anxiety and rebound insomnia have been reported after benzodiazepine cessation, especially with the use of high-potency benzodiazepines with a short to medium elimination half-life.

Persistent Postwithdrawal Disorder

Various symptoms lasting for months or even years following benzodiazepine discontinuation also have been described. Long duration of treatment with benzodiazepines and use of high-potency benzodiazepines with a short to medium elimination half-life may constitute a risk factor for persistent postwithdrawal symptoms (Ashton 1991).

Assessment

Symptoms are assessed through patient reporting or active questioning, physical examination if necessary, and observation of any seizure activity.

Management

The notion that a benzodiazepine must be discontinued, regardless of the context and cost to the patient, should be avoided. Instead, the key task is to make sure that the patient is ready for benzodiazepine discontinuation, which usually means that the patient feels confident enough to cope with the

underlying anxiety or distress without relying on the medication. Slow and individualized tapering of benzodiazepines is
usually used to decrease the risk of withdrawal and rebound
symptoms. However, this risk cannot be entirely eliminated
even with a longer-lasting taper and use of benzodiazepines
that are generally less likely to be implicated in severe withdrawal reactions (e.g., clonazepam). Although benzodiazepines
with a short elimination half-life (e.g., lorazepam) are sometimes replaced during taper by those with a longer elimination
half-life (e.g., diazepam) to prevent or decrease the severity of
withdrawal symptoms, there is no convincing evidence of the
efficacy of this method (e.g., Murphy and Tyrer 1991).

Patients usually benefit from psychoeducation about
benzodiazepine cessation, and cognitive-behavioral therapy
may be useful during the discontinuation process. Some patients may need much more time to complete discontinuation
than others, and the rate at which the taper proceeds should
be adjusted to the needs, concerns, and symptoms of individual patients. The whole discontinuation process bears strik-
ing similarities to the discontinuation of SSRIs and SNRIs.
Management of persistent postwithdrawal disorder depends
on the type and severity of the symptoms.

Follow-Up Management

As is the case with the cessation of all psychotropic medications, there is a risk of relapse following discontinuation of
benzodiazepines. This risk can be mitigated by provision of
support, various psychosocial interventions, or structured
psychological therapy.

Conclusion

Discontinuation of all psychotropic medications carries a risk
of withdrawal or rebound symptoms, and some drugs also
have a relatively low risk of persistent postwithdrawal symptoms. In addition, a proportion of patients may relapse following medication cessation. The exact calculation of these
risks is not possible, although some risk factors carry more
weight than others. It is important to distinguish between
various consequences of medication discontinuation because
of their different implications for management. Withdrawal
symptoms and other symptoms that occur in the aftermath of

medication discontinuation should be neither overemphasized nor underestimated. Relapse is arguably the most important potential consequence of medication cessation. In the absence of evidence-based guidelines for discontinuing psychotropic medications, implementing a slow, individualized taper whenever possible is recommended. This can be achieved only within a framework of a good patient-physician relationship, collaboration, and shared decision-making.

Key Points

Following discontinuation of psychotropic medications, patients may experience withdrawal symptoms, rebound symptoms, persistent postwithdrawal symptoms, or relapse of the condition for which the medication was originally prescribed.

Although a slow, individualized taper does not necessarily prevent untoward events after medication discontinuation, it decreases the risk of these events.

Medication discontinuation should be construed as a collaborative effort that is crucially characterized by flexibility and shared decision-making.

References

Ashton H: Protracted withdrawal syndromes from benzodiazepines. J Subst Abuse Treat 8(1–2):19–28, 1991 1675688

Cerovecki A, Musil R, Klimke A, et al: Withdrawal symptoms and rebound syndromes associated with switching and discontinuing atypical antipsychotics: theoretical background and practical recommendations. CNS Drugs 27(7):545–572, 2013 23821039

Chouinard G, Chouinard V-A: Atypical antipsychotics: CATIE study, drug-induced movement disorder and resulting iatrogenic psychiatric-like symptoms, supersensitivity rebound psychosis and withdrawal discontinuation syndromes. Psychother Psychosom 77(2):69–77, 2008 18230939

Chouinard G, Chouinard V-A: New classification of selective serotonin reuptake inhibitor withdrawal. Psychother Psychosom 84(2):63–71, 2015 25721565

Cosci F, Chouinard G: Acute and persistent withdrawal syndromes following discontinuation of psychotropic medications. Psychother Psychosom 89(5):283–306, 2020 32259826

Davies J, Read J: A systematic review into the incidence, severity and duration of antidepressant withdrawal effects: are guidelines evidence-based? Addict Behav 97:111–121, 2019 30292574

Fava GA, Belaise C: Discontinuing antidepressant drugs: lesson from a failed trial and extensive clinical experience. Psychother Psychosom 87(5):257–267, 2018 30149374

Hengartner MP, Schulthess L, Sorensen A, Framer A: Protracted withdrawal syndrome after stopping antidepressants: a descriptive quantitative analysis of consumer narratives from a large internet forum. Ther Adv Psychopharmacol 10:1–13, 2020 33489088

Horowitz MA, Taylor D: Tapering of SSRI treatment to mitigate withdrawal symptoms. Lancet Psychiatry 6(6):538–546, 2019 30850328

Murphy SM, Tyrer P: A double-blind comparison of the effects of gradual withdrawal of lorazepam, diazepam and bromazepam in benzodiazepine dependence. Br J Psychiatry 158:511–516, 1991 1675901

Chapter 7

Hepatotoxicity of Psychotropic Medications

Ashika Bains, M.D.

The strategy behind choosing psychotropic medication must consider hepatotoxicity, particularly in patients with higher-risk profiles, because medications used in psychiatry and neurology are the second most implicated in drug-induced liver injury in Western countries (Telles-Correia et al. 2017; Todorović Vukotić et al. 2021). Liver injury or hepatotoxicity is defined as damage to the liver as evidenced by elevations in liver function tests (LFTs) greater than or equal to 1.25 times the upper limit of normal results and/or the presence of symptoms of liver disease. In people taking therapeutic doses of medication, the incidence of drug-induced liver injury is between 0.001% and 0.1% (Sedky et al. 2012). Risk factors for drug-induced liver injury include older age, female sex, obesity, pregnancy, alcohol use, genetic polymorphisms, and primary sclerosing cholangitis in post–liver transplant cases (Giordano and Zervos 2013). Children are at increased risk when taking valproate (Maddrey 2013). Drug-induced liver injury can manifest idiosyncratically or as a result of direct hepatotoxicity. Direct toxicity results from hepatocytes generating toxic metabolites; such toxicity has a short latency and is dose dependent, predictable, and reproducible (Pugh et al. 2009; Todorović Vukotić et al. 2021). Idiosyncratic toxicity is dose independent, with possibly a long latency period, and can be subdivided into metabolic and immunologic reactions. Metabolic reactions may result from genetic polymorphisms producing toxic metabolites, whereas immunologic reactions have features of hypersensitivity (Pugh et al. 2009; Sedky et al. 2012). Another type of drug-induced reaction is steatosis, or fat accumulation in the liver.

Recognition and Detection

Drug-induced liver injury can have a broad range of clinical manifestations from asymptomatic enzyme abnormalities to overt liver failure. Biomarkers can assist in determining the type of injury, which includes hepatocellular, cholestatic, and mixed type (Sedky et al. 2012; Telles-Correia et al. 2017). Early symptoms of liver injury include abdominal pain, fatigue, lack of appetite, nausea, vomiting, and fever. Itching or pruritus suggests cholestatic injury. With more severe symptoms, patients may report joint or muscle pain, a tendency to bruise easily, yellowing skin, abdominal swelling, tremors, or disorientation. Immunologic reactions cause hypersensitivity features such as fever and skin reactions. Those with jaundice and high LFTs have the worst prognosis, with an approximately 10%–50% mortality rate (Sedky et al. 2012).

Culprit Medications

Antidepressants

Antidepressant-induced liver injury is generally idiosyncratic with a hepatocellular pattern and an estimated incidence of 0.5%–3.0% for asymptomatic alanine transaminase (ALT) elevation (Bunchorntavakul and Reddy 2017; Todorović Vukotić et al. 2021). In general, selective serotonin reuptake inhibitors (SSRIs) and serotonin-norepinephrine reuptake inhibitors (SNRIs) are less likely to cause hepatotoxicity compared with monoamine oxidase inhibitors (MAOIs) and tricyclic antidepressants (TCAs). Higher-risk agents include amitriptyline, imipramine, and nefazodone (available only in generic form in the United States). There have been reports of severe liver injury with venlafaxine, duloxetine, sertraline, bupropion, and trazodone. Lower-risk agents include citalopram, escitalopram, fluvoxamine, desvenlafaxine, and selegiline.

For SSRIs, the agents most associated with LFT elevations three times the upper limit of normal results are sertraline and paroxetine, with an approximate incidence of 1%. Fluoxetine, citalopram, and escitalopram have the least risk, with an approximate incidence of less than 1% (Bunchorntavakul and Reddy 2017; Sedky et al. 2012). Cases of mixed-type and cholestatic injury have been described with fluoxetine (National Institutes of Health 2021). There are some reported cases of severe toxicity with sertraline (Sedky et al. 2012). There have not been any reports of fulminant liver failure with citalopram and escitalopram (Bunchorntavakul and Reddy 2017; Sedky et al. 2012). Fluvoxamine has been linked to sporadic instances of hepatotoxicity.

For SNRIs, the medication most associated with LFT elevations three times the upper limit of normal results is duloxetine, which is associated with hepatocellular, cholestatic, and mixed-type liver injury. Duloxetine should be avoided or used with caution in patients with evidence of chronic liver disease, substantial alcohol use, or higher susceptibility to drug-induced liver injury (Bunchorntavakul and Reddy 2017; Sedky et al. 2012; Todorović Vukotić et al. 2021). The incidence of venlafaxine-induced ALT elevations three times the upper limit of normal results is low. Desvenlafaxine is associated with rare hepatic enzyme elevation when used in high doses (Bunchorntavakul and Reddy 2017; Sedky et al. 2012).

For alternative antidepressants, nefazodone has three to four times the risk of liver failure compared with similar drugs and carries an FDA black box warning for hepatotoxicity (Sedky et al. 2012; Selim and Kaplowitz 1999; Todorović Vukotić et al. 2021). Trazodone generally does not cause hepatotoxicity, although some cases have been reported (Sedky et al. 2012; Selim and Kaplowitz 1999). Bupropion has rarely been associated with drug-induced liver injury. Mirtazapine was generally considered safe, with sporadic cases of hepatotoxicity after long-term exposure (Sedky et al. 2012). Nevertheless, a recent retrospective study from Germany found that mirtazapine was one of the prescribed antidepressants associated with the occurrence of elevated liver enzymes (Ueberberg et al. 2020).

For MAOIs, phenelzine and tranylcypromine have been associated with hepatic damage (Sedky et al. 2012). Selegiline has not been associated with hepatic damage. For TCAs, imipramine can induce nonprogressive cholestatic jaundice and cross-reactivity with other tricyclics (Selim and Kaplowitz 1999).

Lastly, certain SSRIs can contribute to drug-induced liver injury by elevating levels of other medications via inhibition of cytochrome enzymes. Fluoxetine, paroxetine, fluvoxamine, and, to a lesser extent, sertraline can inhibit cytochrome isoform 2D6. Fluvoxamine can also inhibit 1A2 and 3A4, potentially raising clozapine and aripiprazole levels, respectively (Todorović Vukotić et al. 2021).

Hepatotoxicity of Psychotropic Medications   **65**

Antipsychotics

Antipsychotic medications have frequently been associated with benign, transient LFT elevations (Sedky et al. 2012; Selim and Kaplowitz 1999; Telles-Correia et al. 2017). Antipsychotics include first-generation agents (FGAs) and second-generation agents (SGAs). Although SGAs have lower cases of associated drug-induced liver injury, they do have the potential to induce metabolic syndrome and subsequent steatosis. Higher-risk agents include chlorpromazine and other phenothiazines, clozapine, and quetiapine. Lower-risk agents include aripiprazole, ziprasidone, paliperidone, and lurasidone.

For FGAs, phenothiazines (chlorpromazine, fluphenazine, perphenazine, prochlorperazine, thioridazine, trifluoperazine) have an estimated incidence of asymptomatic LFT abnormalities in up to 20% of patients and overt liver disease in up to 1%, with features of hypersensitivity in about half of the cases (Sedky et al. 2012; Selim and Kaplowitz 1999). Severe drug-induced liver injury has been reported for chlorpromazine (Todorović Vukotić et al. 2021). Chlorpromazine toxicity appears to be idiosyncratic with reported cases of progression to cirrhosis. Cross-reactivity with other phenothiazines is rare. Butyrophenones (droperidol, haloperidol) have a rare incidence of hepatotoxicity. The incidence of LFTs more than three times the upper limit of normal results with haloperidol is 2.4% (Sedky et al. 2012; Selim and Kaplowitz 1999).

For SGAs, clozapine is the agent most associated with hepatotoxicity, with asymptomatic LFT increases that are often transient in up to 60% of patients. There are several case reports of fulminant failure with clozapine at moderate doses, and clozapine can inhibit multiple cytochrome enzyme isoforms, contributing to accumulation of other hepatotoxic medications (Todorović Vukotić et al. 2021). There may be cross hepatotoxicity between clozapine and olanzapine. In patients prescribed olanzapine, cases of drug-induced liver injury with hepatocellular and cholestatic patterns have been reported, with resolution within 4 weeks of discontinuation in most cases (Slim et al. 2016). Risperidone has been associated with severe LFT elevations, whereas paliperidone is excreted mainly through the kidneys and has no known toxic metabolites (Sedky et al. 2012; Todorović Vukotić et al. 2021). Cross hepatotoxicity may exist with use of risperidone and quetiapine. Quetiapine has been associated with cholestasis and rare fulminant hepatic failure; therefore, small dose increases are advised for hepatically compromised individuals (Sedky et al. 2012; Todorović Vukotić et al. 2021). In rare instances, ziprasidone has been associated with drug rash with eosinophilia and systemic symptoms (Bunchorntavakul and Reddy 2017; Slim et al. 2016). Aripiprazole is associated with fewer abnormalities.

A recent observational study in Germany reported an overall rate of severe antipsychotic-related drug-induced liver injury of 0.07%. In terms of rates of severe injury related to use of single antipsychotics, olanzapine was found to have the highest event rate, followed by clozapine, with first-generation medications such as levomepromazine and promethazine ranking fourth and fifth, respectively (Druschky et al. 2021).

Mood Stabilizers

Generally, newer-generation mood stabilizers are better tolerated and carry a lower risk of hepatotoxicity than older agents (Kamitaki et al. 2021). Valproate is associated with transient elevations of aminotransferases, hyperbilirubinemia, steatosis, and rare hypersensitivity reactions with a latency up to 2 years (Sedky et al. 2012; Telles-Correia et al. 2017). Valproate is also associated with hyperammonemic encephalopathy and polycystic ovarian disease and might be related to hepatocellular adenoma. The total incidence of drug-induced liver injury due to carbamazepine is about 1%. However, a recent study reported that an OR of any degree of drug-induced liver injury associated with carbamazepine exceeded their report of valproate (Kamitaki et al. 2021). Some cases of hypersensitivity syndrome within the first 8 weeks of carbamazepine treatment have been reported. Carbamazepine is associated with hyperammonemia and Stevens-Johnson syndrome (Sedky et al. 2012; Telles-Correia et al. 2017). Oxcarbazepine may have a safer profile. Lamotrigine causes elevations in LFTs in 1% of patients and has been associated with major hypersensitivity reactions (Stevens-Johnson syndrome, toxic epidermal necrolysis). Risk factors include younger age, rapid escalation of dose, and concomitant use of valproate, which can increase lamotrigine levels by 200% (Bunchorntavakul and Reddy 2017; Telles-Correia et al. 2017). Levetiracetam is renally excreted and is associated with asymptomatic ALT elevation but not hepatitis. Topiramate is excreted mainly by the kidneys, although it causes LFT elevations in 1% of patients (Sedky et al. 2012; Telles-Correia et al. 2017). Long-term lithium use can induce LFT abnormalities, which are generally temporary and asymptomatic.

Benzodiazepines and Nonbenzodiazepine Receptor Agonists

Benzodiazepine-induced liver damage is rare, with a few cases of cholestatic reaction associated with diazepam, chlordiazepoxide, and flurazepam. Lorazepam, oxazepam, and temazepam have not been associated with liver injury (Sedky et al. 2012; Selim and Kaplowitz 1999; Telles-Correia et al. 2017). A recent study of individuals taking high doses (defined as the equivalent of 50 mg of diazepam) for at least 6 months did not find severe drug-induced liver injury (Lugoboni et al. 2018). Gabapentin and pregabalin are mainly excreted by the kidneys, and adverse effects on the liver are rare.

Miscellaneous Agents

Tacrine has been associated with fatal liver damage, with nearly all tacrine-induced toxicity occurring in the first 12 weeks of treatment (Sedky et al. 2012; Selim and Kaplowitz 1999). Donepezil, rivastigmine, memantine, and galantamine have rarely been associated with drug-induced liver injury. Methadone, particularly with concurrent alcohol use, has been linked to cases of hepatotoxicity (Sedky et al. 2012). Buprenorphine-induced liver injury is rare. Naltrexone has been associated with hepatotoxicity in doses greater than recommended and is contraindicated in individuals with hepatitis (Sedky et al. 2012). There is no evidence of buspirone-induced liver toxicity. Prazosin is generally considered safe. Four years of postmarketing research has identified three cases of hepatotoxicity with atomoxetine (Sedky et al. 2012).

Assessment

Recognizing drug-induced liver injury can pose a diagnostic challenge because of confounding factors (alcohol use, weight, herbal supplements, medical comorbidities) and the latency period of idiosyncratic reactions. An accurate diagnosis relies on establishing a temporal relationship and excluding alternative causes of liver injury. An initial assessment should include a thorough history of substance use, the time of initiation of potential hepatotoxic medications, and the onset and course of symptoms. Special attention should be paid to medication interactions that may result in increased plasma levels of a hepatotoxic drug.

Physical examination findings can range in severity from hepatitis to cirrhosis. Initial findings include abdominal pain (generalized or specific to the right upper quadrant), fatigue, emesis, and anorexia. Progressive disease findings include jaundice, pruritus, ascites, asterixis, tremor, purpura, and encephalopathy. Those with drug-induced hypersensitivity may present with fever, facial edema, and cutaneous eruptions.

Laboratory studies alone cannot be used to diagnose drug-induced liver injury but may assist in identification of the type of injury, which would guide treatment. Liver function can be measured by using aminotransferases (ALT, aspartate transaminase [AST]), bilirubin, alkaline phosphatase (ALP), albumin, and coagulation tests. Hepatocellular injury is associated with elevations in ALT, no change in ALP, and, in severe cases, an increase in bilirubin (Garcia-Cortes et al. 2020; Giordano and Zervos 2013; Telles-Correia et al. 2017; Watkins 2013). Cholestatic injury is associated with elevated ALP at least two times the upper limit of normal results or an ALT-to-ALP ratio of less than 2 with both ALT and ALP greater than the upper limit of normal results, suggesting injury to the bile ducts (Garcia-Cortes et al. 2020; Giordano and Zervos 2013; Sedky et al. 2012; Telles-Correia et al. 2017). With mixed-type injury, both ALP and ALT are increased. In general, increases in LFT greater than three times the upper limit of normal results carry the greatest risk. Steatosis reactions can be measured with elevations in LFTs, fasting blood sugar, hemoglobin A1c, and lipid profile and with visualization of fat accumulation in the liver via ultrasound or CT scan.

In the assessment of drug-induced liver injury, exclusion of alternative causes of liver injury should be pursued. A differential diagnosis includes viral hepatitis, autoimmune hepatitis, alcoholic hepatitis, Wilson's disease, biliary disease, hemochromatosis, and vascular disease affecting the portal vein. Screening for viral or autoimmune etiology via blood work and using imaging (ultrasound, CT scan) can help exclude alternative causes of injury.

Management

Particularly in those patients at high risk for drug-induced hepatotoxicity, baseline LFTs should be assessed prior to initiating psychotropic medications. In addition, a list of current medications should be obtained, and polypharmacy should be minimized, if possible. In the absence of concern, both LFTs and metabolic parameters should be monitored annually.

If drug-induced liver injury is suspected and laboratory analysis indicates an increase in aminotransferases less than three times the upper limit of normal results, LFTs should be monitored more frequently. If asymptomatic elevation of LFTs persists, a decrease in dose or discontinuation of medication should be considered.

If an increase in aminotransferases greater than three times the upper limit of normal results occurs and/or the patient is clinically symptomatic, the offending medication should be discontinued, and biomarkers should be monitored. If autoimmune hepatitis or a cholestatic pattern of injury occurs, corticosteroids should be administered. Pruritus can be treated with emollients, diphenhydramine, or bile acid resins.

If fulminant hepatic failure is suspected, as evidenced by severe symptoms such as encephalopathy and severe laboratory abnormalities such as thrombocytopenia and prolonged prothrombin time, the patient should be transferred to the intensive care unit and treated for sequelae of liver failure.

Follow-Up Management

If medications must be discontinued, the patient should be carefully monitored until symptoms resolve and LFTs return to baseline levels. Patients with severe disease should avoid alcohol use, fatty foods, undercooked meats, and hepatotoxic medications. Liver damage generally resolves after discontinuation of medication and reappears with pharmaceutical rechallenge. Patients with severe disease or hypersensitivity reactions should not be rechallenged. Patients with mild injury can be rechallenged with a lower dose or slower titration if alternative medication is not available. Overall, when rechallenging the patient leads to additional liver dysfunction, symptoms occur more rapidly with a similar or less severe pattern compared with the initial injury (Papay et al. 2009). Potential negative health consequences of drug rechallenge in patients with previous drug-induced liver injury should be thoroughly discussed before reinitiation of medication. Finally, cross-reactivity should be considered when choosing alternative agents.

Conclusion

All psychotropic medications have the potential for hepatotoxicity. Clinicians are tasked with identifying at-risk populations and tracking the association between drug initiation and laboratory abnormalities or symptoms. History, physical examination, and laboratory studies can help identify drug-induced liver injury and exclude alternative causes of liver injury. Management may necessitate discontinuation of the offending agent and initiation of treatment for liver disease.

Key Points

Hepatotoxicity is defined as liver function test elevations greater than or equal to 1.25 times the upper limit of normal results and/or the presence of symptoms of liver injury.

Drug-induced liver injury can manifest as direct hepatotoxicity idiosyncratically, with patterns of injury occurring as hepatocellular, cholestatic, or mixed-type injury or steatosis.

Selective serotonin reuptake inhibitors and serotonin-norepinephrine reuptake inhibitors are less likely to cause hepatotoxicity than monoamine oxidase inhibitors and tricyclic antidepressants.

Second-generation agents have a lower risk of drug-induced liver injury compared with first-generation agents, although some can produce steatosis.

Newer-generation mood stabilizers carry less risk of hepatotoxicity than older agents.

If liver function tests are greater than three times the upper limit of normal results and/or the patient has symptoms of liver dysfunction, offending medications should be discontinued.

Liver damage generally resolves after discontinuation of medication and reoccurs with rechallenge.

References

Bunchorntavakul C, Reddy KR: Drug hepatotoxicity: newer agents. Clin Liver Dis 21(1):115–134, 2017 27842767

Druschky K, Toto S, Bleich S, et al: Severe drug-induced liver injury in patients under treatment with antipsychotic drugs: data from the AMSP study. World J Biol Psychiatry 22(5):373–386, 2021 32892689

Garcia-Cortes M, Robles-Diaz M, Stephens C, et al: Drug induced liver injury: an update. Arch Toxicol 94(10):3381–3407, 2020 32852569

Giordano CM, Zervos XB: Clinical manifestations and treatment of drug-induced hepatotoxicity. Clin Liver Dis 17(4):565–573, viii, 2013 24099018

Kamitaki BK, Minacapelli CD, Zhang P, et al: Drug-induced liver injury associated with antiseizure medications from the FDA Adverse Event Reporting System (FAERS). Epilepsy Behav 117:107832, 2021 33626490

Lugoboni F, Mirijello A, Morbioli L, et al: Does high-dose benzodiazepine abuse really produce liver toxicity? Results from a series of 201 benzodiazepine monoabusers. Expert Opin Drug Saf 17(5):451–456, 2018 29621907

Maddrey WC: Clinical manifestations and management of drug-induced liver diseases, in Drug-Induced Liver Disease. Edited by Kaplowitz N, DeLeve LD. New York, Academic Press, 2013, pp 229–240

National Institutes of Health: LiverTox: clinical and research information on drug-induced liver injury. National Institute of Diabetes and Digestive and Kidney Diseases, 2021. Available at: https://www.ncbi.nlm.nih.gov/books/NBK547852. Accessed July 7, 2022.

Papay JI, Clines D, Rafi R, et al: Drug-induced liver injury following positive drug rechallenge. Regul Toxicol Pharmacol 54(1):84–90, 2009 19303041

Pugh AJ, Barve AJ, Falkner K, et al: Drug-induced hepatotoxicity or drug-induced liver injury. Clin Liver Dis 13(2):277–294, 2009 19442919

Sedky K, Nazir R, Joshi A, et al: Which psychotropic medications induce hepatotoxicity? Gen Hosp Psychiatry 34(1):53–61, 2012 22133982

Selim K, Kaplowitz N: Hepatotoxicity of psychotropic drugs. Hepatology 29(5):1347–1351, 1999 10216114

Slim M, Medina-Caliz I, Gonzalez-Jimenez A, et al: Hepatic safety of atypical antipsychotics: current evidence and future directions. Drug Saf 39(10):925–943, 2016 27449495

Telles-Correia D, Barbosa A, Cortez-Pinto H, et al: Psychotropic drugs and liver disease: a critical review of pharmacokinetics and liver toxicity. World J Gastrointest Pharmacol Ther 8(1):26–38, 2017 28217372

Todorović Vukotić N, Dordević J, Pejić S, et al: Antidepressants- and antipsychotics-induced hepatotoxicity. Arch Toxicol 95(3):767–789, 2021 33398419

Ueberberg B, Frommberger U, Messer T, et al: Drug-induced liver injury (DILI) in patients with depression treated with antidepressants: a retrospective multicenter study. Pharmacopsychiatry 53(2):60–64, 2020 31958850

Watkins PB: Biomarkers for drug-induced liver injury, in Drug-Induced Liver Disease. Edited by Kaplowitz N, DeLeve LD. New York, Academic Press, 2013, pp 275–286

Chapter 8

Hypertensive Crisis Associated With Monoamine Oxidase Inhibitors

Mary K. Morreale, M.D.

Monoamine oxidase inhibitors (MAOIs) have been shown to be effective in the treatment of depression, including atypical and treatment-resistant depression, panic disorder, and social anxiety disorder (Krishnan 2007). Because of concerns related to food and drug interactions, this class of medications is not commonly prescribed (Shulman et al. 2009). The mechanism of action of MAOIs is inhibition of monoamine oxidase subtypes MAO-A and MAO-B. MAO-A is primarily found in the brain, intestine, liver, and skin and is responsible for the degradation of serotonin, norepinephrine, dopamine, and dietary tyramine. MAO-B is found in the brain, platelets, and lymphocytes and is active in the breakdown of dopamine and tyramine. MAOIs bind to MAO enzymes and prevent the degradation of the substances mentioned, leading to increased amounts in the synaptic cleft. MAO-A inhibition is necessary for antidepressant efficacy, which is thought to be mediated not by increased synaptic serotonin, norepinephrine, and dopamine but rather by presynaptic and postsynaptic activity (Krishnan 2007).

The FDA has approved four MAOIs for psychiatric treatment: isocarboxazid, phenelzine, tranylcypromine, and selegiline. The first three are nonselective, indicating inhibition of both subtypes of MAO. The latter, selegiline, approved in a transdermal patch, specifically inhibits MAO-B below the dosage of 6 mg every 24 hours but becomes nonselective at dosages of 9 mg every 24 hours and greater (Somerset Pharmaceuticals 2014). All MAOIs available in the United States are irreversible and therefore bind to the MAO enzyme permanently. A minimum of 7–10 days is required for enzyme regeneration and subsequent return to baseline functioning of amine degradation. Reversible inhibitors of MAO-A (RIMAs) are available outside the United States and can be displaced from the MAO enzyme by competitive inhibitors (Lum and Stahl 2012). For this reason, RIMAs have less significant dietary and drug restrictions.

When dietary tyramine is ingested, it is typically metabolized by MAO in the liver and gut. When a patient takes a nonselective and irreversible MAOI, this degradation is blocked. In this circumstance, tyramine enters adrenergic nerve terminals, where it displaces already elevated levels of stored norepinephrine. When this excess norepinephrine enters the sympathetic nervous system, vasoconstriction and hypertension ensue. A similar reaction occurs when a patient taking a nonselective and irreversible MAOI ingests sympathomimetic medications such as phenylephrine and pseudoephedrine, which are commonly included in over-the-counter cold and cough preparations. Chronic treatment with MAOIs increases the risk of hypertension, as does the potency of the MAOI, rate of gastric emptying, and dose of both the MAOI and the offending agent (Gillman 2018). Unless large amounts of tyramine are ingested (more than 100 mg), hypertension tends to be transient (Gillman 2018).

Hypertensive emergency is defined as a sudden increase in blood pressure greater than 180 mm Hg systolic and 110 mm Hg diastolic associated with acute end-organ injury in the cerebrovascular, cardiovascular, ophthalmologic, hematologic, and renovascular systems (Miller et al. 2020). In patients prescribed nonselective and irreversible MAOIs, a hypertensive emergency can occur when dietary tyramine and sympathomimetic medications are ingested.

Recognition and Detection

Clinical symptoms of hypertensive emergency reflect the organ system affected. The most common types of hypertensive emergencies are ischemic and hemorrhagic cerebral vascular accident and acute heart failure (Miller et al. 2020). Patients with ischemic stroke can present with focal neurological findings and altered mental status. Those with hemorrhagic stroke can present with headache and vomiting. Patients in acute heart failure may experience shortness of breath, tachypnea, and palpitations, and those with myocardial infarction may experience chest pain. On rare occasions, patients with hypertensive encephalopathy can develop fresh flame hemorrhages, papilledema, and exudates on direct funduscopic examination.

Culprit Medications, Illegal Drugs, and Foods

Medications and illegal drugs associated with MAOI hypertensive crisis include stimulants, sympathomimetics used for local and general anesthesia, ephedrine, oxymetazoline, phenylephrine, phentermine, pseudoephedrine, and cocaine. Foods that contain tyramine include aged cheese; meat, poultry, or fish that is aged, cured, improperly stored, or spoiled; overripe or spoiled fruits and vegetables, broad bean pods (fava beans), and banana peel; soy sauce, tofu, and soybean condiments; concentrated yeast extract; some draft beers; and fermented foods.

Assessment

Historically, patients taking MAOIs were prescribed oral chlorpromazine or nifedipine and advised to take this medication in an outpatient setting if severe headache, which is one indication of hypertension, developed (Cockhill and Remick 1987). Given the risk for the rapid development of hypotension with this practice, it is no longer recommended, and patients with suspicion of MAOI-associated hypertension are advised to go to an emergency department setting for treatment (Cockhill and Remick 1987). A rapid reduction of blood pressure can be detrimental in certain circumstances, such as ischemic stroke, in which further hypoperfusion could cause additional neurological damage. Therefore, end-organ damage must be evaluated before initiating hypertensive treatment.

In patients presenting to the emergency department with a marked elevation of blood pressure (>180 mm Hg systolic and 110 mm Hg diastolic) associated with MAOI treatment, an examination of end-organ damage must occur. This includes a basic metabolic panel, complete blood count, urinalysis, electrocardiogram, and chest X-ray. Depending on symptom presentation, an additional workup might include assessment of biomarkers for cardiac injury, including troponin and natriuretic peptides; CT angiography of the thorax and abdomen; CT or MRI of the brain; and ophthalmologic examination (Miller et al. 2020).

Management

If no evidence of end-organ injury is seen, the current paradigm of management does not recommend antihypertensive treatment (Krishnan 2007). If evidence of end-organ damage is found, as described in the systems mentioned in the previous "Assessment" section, treatment with the intravenous α-adrenergic blocker phentolamine should begin. If this is ineffective, nicardipine and clevidipine, which are short-acting calcium channel blockers, are indicated (Miller et al. 2020).

Dosing of these medications varies. For phentolamine, the initial dose is a 1–15 mg IV bolus followed by a 1–40 mg/hour infusion until target blood pressure is reached (Miller et al. 2020). The initial dose infusion of clevidipine is 1–2 mg/hour. Titration occurs by doubling the dose at short (90-second) intervals until goal blood pressure is approached. When this occurs, the dose is decreased to less than double, and the interval of infusion is lengthened to 5–10 minutes. Increasing the infusion by 1–2 mg/hour leads to an approximate decrease of 2–4 mm Hg in systolic pressure, and most patients respond to 4–6 mg/hour. The maximum dose is 16 mg/hour (Chiesi 2021). Finally, the dose of nicardipine is 5–15 mg/hour (Miller et al. 2020).

Follow-Up Management

Following treatment to reduce acute hypertension, a nutritional consultation is recommended to educate the patient about dietary requirements when taking MAOIs. In addition, a thorough conversation about concurrent medications to avoid must occur prior to discharge.

Conclusion

Given the low rates of MAOI prescriptions, an associated hypertensive emergency is likely a rare phenomenon. If it is suspected, patients should be advised to go to an emergency department where blood pressure and potential end-organ damage can be adequately assessed. If end-organ damage exists, treatment with phentolamine, nicardipine, or clevidipine is warranted.

Key Points

Hypertensive emergency is defined as a sudden increase in blood pressure greater than 180 mm Hg systolic and 110 mm Hg diastolic associated with acute end-organ injury.

When a patient who is taking a monoamine oxidase inhibitor ingests either dietary tyramine or a sympathomimetic medication, hypertensive emergency can occur.

Patients with markedly elevated blood pressure resulting from a combination of a monoamine oxidase inhibitor and dietary tyramine or sympathomimetic medications should be assessed in an emergency department setting.

Unless end-organ damage is present, treatment with antihypertensive medications is not warranted.

If evidence of end-organ damage is found, patients should initially receive phentolamine, followed by nicardipine or clevidipine.

Those patients who present with hypertension associated with monoamine oxidase inhibitor treatment should receive a nutritional consultation to review dietary restrictions and should take part in a thorough discussion of contraindicated medications.

References

Chiesi: Dosing and administration guide for Cleviprex (clevidipine) injectable emulsion. April 2021. Available at: https://resources.chiesiusa.com/Cleviprex/CLEVIPREX_Dosing_and_Administration_Fact_Sheet.pdf. Accessed July 7, 2022.

Cockhill LA, Remick RA: Blood pressure effects of monoamine oxidase inhibitors—the highs and lows. Can J Psychiatry 32(9):803–808, 1987 2893660

Gillman PK: A reassessment of the safety profile of monoamine oxidase inhibitors: elucidating tired old tyramine myths. J Neural Transm (Vienna) 125(11):1707–1717, 2018 30255284

Krishnan KR: Revisiting monoamine oxidase inhibitors. J Clin Psychiatry 68(Suppl 8):35–41, 2007 17640156

Lum CT, Stahl SM: Opportunities for reversible inhibitors of monoamine oxidase-A (RIMAs) in the treatment of depression. CNS Spectr 17(3):107–120, 2012 23888494

Miller J, McNaughton C, Joyce K, et al: Hypertension management in emergency departments. Am J Hypertens 33(10):927–934, 2020 32307541

Shulman KI, Fischer HD, Herrmann N, et al: Current prescription patterns and safety profile of irreversible monoamine oxidase inhibitors: a population-based cohort study of older adults. J Clin Psychiatry 70(12):1681–1686, 2009 19852903

Somerset Pharmaceuticals: Emsam: highlights of prescribing information. September 2014. Available at: www.accessdata.fda.gov/drugsatfda_docs/label/2014/021336s005s010,021708s000lbl.pdf. Accessed July 7, 2022.

Chapter 9

Hyponatremia, Especially in Older Adults

Art Walaszek, M.D.

Hyponatremia, defined as a serum sodium concentration below 135 mEq/L, is the most common electrolyte disorder in clinical practice (Verbalis et al. 2013). Maintaining normal serum sodium concentration depends on the functioning of antidiuretic hormone (ADH, also known as vasopressin). When plasma osmolality is high (indicating dehydration) or plasma volume is low (indicating volume depletion), ADH is released. ADH binds to vasopressin V_2 receptors in the distal tubules of the kidneys, resulting in resorption of water from urine back into the bloodstream (Verbalis et al. 2013). When plasma osmolality is low, ADH is suppressed, which allows the kidneys to excrete more dilute urine by preventing absorption of water from urine; thus, individuals can maintain a normal concentration of sodium (Verbalis et al. 2013).

Unfortunately, as people age, their kidneys become less able to dilute urine. Furthermore, many medications may prevent suppression of ADH release, stimulate ADH release, or increase the sensitivity of the kidneys to ADH (Jacob and Spinler 2006). Older adults, especially women, are at risk for developing the syndrome of inappropriate antidiuretic hormone secretion (SIADH) and hyponatremia. Older adults are thought to be at higher risk for hyponatremia because of lower body mass, lower volume of distribution, decreased renal clearance, and polypharmacy (Pinkhasov et al. 2021). Risk factors for antidepressant-induced hyponatremia include age 65 or older, female sex, use of a diuretic medication (11–13 times increased risk), re-

_____
I thank Tripti Singh, M.D., Department of Medicine, University of Wisconsin School of Medicine and Public Health, for her guidance and for her review of the chapter.

cent history of pneumonia, low body weight, lower baseline sodium concentration (<138 mEq/L), liver disease, and history of hyponatremia (Gandhi et al. 2017; Jacob and Spinler 2006).

Hyponatremia is associated with many adverse outcomes, including delirium, falls, fractures, seizures, hospitalization, and death (Jacob and Spinler 2006; Verbalis et al. 2013). Three very large retrospective studies of older adults in Ontario, Canada, provided estimates for the risk of hospitalization for hyponatremia due to psychotropic medications. The 30-day risk of hospitalization was 0.33% for antidepressants, about 5 times higher than the risk in the control group (Gandhi et al. 2017); for carbamazepine, it was 0.39%, about 8 times higher than in the control group (Gandhi et al. 2016a); and for antipsychotics, it was 0.15%, about 1.6 times higher than in the control group (Gandhi et al. 2016b). Hyponatremia, especially when chronic, increases the risk for gait instability, falls, osteoporosis, and fractures among older adults (Verbalis et al. 2013). Hyponatremia is associated with increased mortality in people with heart failure, in people with liver disease, and among medical inpatients (Verbalis et al. 2013).

Recognition and Detection

Clinicians should have a low index of suspicion for hyponatremia in older adults, especially in older women and older adults who are taking a diuretic. I recommend checking serum sodium concentration before starting an antidepressant, carbamazepine, or oxcarbazepine in any patient with risk factors for hyponatremia, especially older age (65 and older), female sex, and current use of a thiazide diuretic. I also recommend considering checking sodium concentration prior to starting other antiepileptic drugs and antipsychotic medications. The American Geriatrics Society Beers Criteria for Potentially Inappropriate Medication Use in Older Adults offer no specific recommendations beyond "monitor[ing] sodium level closely when starting or changing dosages in older adults" (2019 American Geriatrics Society Beers Criteria® Update Expert Panel 2019, p. 13).

For those patients at risk for hyponatremia who have normal sodium levels at baseline, I recommend rechecking sodium concentration 2 weeks after starting the medication, 2 weeks after each titration, and periodically afterward. Note that sodium concentration may decline, even if frank hyponatremia does not develop.

I recommend checking sodium concentration in any patient who is taking a psychotropic medication who develops confusion or gait imbalance. Patients with hyponatremia also may present with nonspecific symptoms such as headache, fatigue, nausea, or vomiting, so clinicians should consider checking sodium concentration in such patients as well (Jacob and Spinler 2006; Verbalis et al. 2013).

For asymptomatic patients without a history of hyponatremia who are taking an antidepressant, antiepileptic drug, or antipsychotic, I recommend checking sodium concentration when they turn 60 years old, if they are prescribed another medication that can cause hyponatremia (e.g., diuretics), and if they develop comorbidities such as heart failure, renal disease, or liver disease.

Culprit Medications and Other Causes

Older adults are especially prone to developing hyponatremia when taking certain medications. The American Geriatrics Society Beers Criteria for Potentially Inappropriate Medication Use in Older Adults list the following medications that may "exacerbate or cause SIADH or hyponatremia": selective serotonin reuptake inhibitors (SSRIs), serotonin-norepinephrine reuptake inhibitors (SNRIs), mirtazapine, tricyclic antidepressants, carbamazepine, oxcarbazepine, antipsychotics, tramadol, desmopressin, and diuretics (2019 American Geriatrics Society Beers Criteria® Update Expert Panel 2019, p. 13). There are case reports of hyponatremia with benzodiazepines, amphetamine/methylphenidate, atomoxetine, and dextromethorphan (Pinkhasov et al. 2021), but the risk is likely very low. Cholinesterase inhibitors and memantine do not appear to be associated with hyponatremia (Pinkhasov et al. 2021). Diuretics, especially thiazides, are the most common cause of medication-induced hyponatremia, including in older adults (Liamis et al. 2008). Other nonpsychotropic medications that can cause hyponatremia include nonsteroidal anti-inflammatory drugs and anticancer drugs (e.g., vincristine, cisplatin, cyclophosphamide) (Liamis et al. 2008).

Antidepressants

Among psychotropic medications, antidepressants have the most extensive literature regarding their propensity to cause hyponatremia. Antidepressants may have effects on ADH release or renal responsiveness to ADH via serotonergic or noradrenergic mechanisms (Jacob and Spinler 2006). Estimates of the incidence of antidepressant-induced hyponatremia range from 0.06% to 40% (De Picker et al. 2014). The only prospective clinical trial that specifically assessed the risk of hyponatremia in older adults taking an antidepressant found that 12% developed hyponatremia with paroxetine, with median time to onset of 9 days (range=1–14 days) (Fabian et al. 2004). A 10-year prospective pharmacovigilance study found that antidepressants were the second most common cause of severe hyponatremia (<116 mEq/L), after thiazide diuretics (Ramírez et al. 2019). There are case reports of bupropion causing hyponatremia, but it appears that the risk is lower than with other antidepressants; in fact, bupropion may be a safe alternative when patients develop hyponatremia with other antidepressants (De Picker et al. 2014). Mirtazapine also may be less likely than SSRIs to cause hyponatremia (Gandhi et al. 2017).

Some patients prescribed an antidepressant may have a decline in sodium concentration without developing hyponatremia. In a prospective study of fluoxetine for depression, the mean sodium concentration among older adults (age 55 and older) decreased from 139.8 to 138.4 mEq/L after 1 week and to 135.2 mEq/L after 3 weeks (Shakibaei et al. 2010). Younger adults (ages 15–35 years) had a much smaller decrease: from 141.6 mEq/L at baseline to 140.8 mEq/L at 3 weeks (Shakibaei et al. 2010). In this study, the incidence of hyponatremia among older adults was 4.7% at 1 week and 15.8% at 3 weeks (Shakibaei et al. 2010).

Hyponatremia typically arises within the first 2 weeks of starting or titrating a medication. As noted earlier, the median time to onset in a prospective study of paroxetine was 9 days after starting the medication, with all cases arising within 14 days (Fabian et al. 2004). Sodium concentration returns to normal levels typically within 2 weeks after stopping the offending medication, although it may take as long as 6 weeks (Jacob and Spinler 2006; Liamis et al. 2008). Hyponatremia is likely to recur following rechallenge with the same medication and perhaps even with a medication of the same class, such as another SSRI (Jacob and Spinler 2006).

Antiepileptic Drugs

Carbamazepine may cause hyponatremia by increasing ADH release. The incidence of carbamazepine-induced hyponatremia is between 4.8% and 41.5%, and the incidence may be even higher with oxcarbazepine (Liamis et al. 2008). In a prospective study of 1,370 people with epilepsy who were treated with carbamazepine or oxcarbazepine, 410 developed hyponatremia; 65% of those with hyponatremia were symptomatic; the risk of symptomatic hyponatremia was higher with oxcarbazepine than with carbamazepine (Berghuis et al. 2021). The risk of hyponatremia correlates with baseline sodium concentration (lower concentration leads to higher risk), carbamazepine dose, and serum carbamazepine level (Liamis et al. 2008). Valproate and topiramate may also cause hyponatremia, although less frequently than carbamazepine (Gandhi et al. 2016a).

Antipsychotics

Long-term use of antipsychotics may cause hyponatremia via supersensitivity of dopamine D_2 receptors, which results in increased ADH levels (Yang and Cheng 2017). Although the incidence of hyponatremia due to antipsychotics is unclear, it appears that first-generation antipsychotics are more likely to cause hyponatremia than are second-generation antipsychotics (Gandhi et al. 2016b; Yang and Cheng 2017). Persons who have tolerated an antipsychotic for years could develop hyponatremia as they age or when they develop medical comorbidities (Yang and Cheng 2017).

Psychogenic Polydipsia

Medications are not the only cause of hyponatremia in people with mental illness. Psychogenic polydipsia can also cause hyponatremia: a person drinks so much water that it overwhelms the person's ability to dilute their urine (Liamis et al. 2008). The psychiatric diagnosis most often associated with psychogenic polydipsia is schizophrenia. An estimated 6%–17% of people with chronic, severe mental illness have psychogenic polydipsia (Illowsky and Kirch 1988). In a study of outpatients with severe mental illness, 16% of whom had polydipsia, the mean daily fluid intake was 4.6 L among those with polydipsia, compared with 2.8 L among those without polydipsia (Iftene et al. 2013). The prevalence of psychogenic polydipsia among older adults is unknown. Another possibility is that a person could be drinking fluids excessively to try to address dry mouth, perhaps caused by psychotropic medications (Liamis et al. 2008). Risk of recurrence is high: in a small prospective study of people hospitalized with psychogenic polydipsia, 52% were readmitted for hyponatremia within a year (Sailer et al. 2017).

Assessment

The assessment of hyponatremia may include checking plasma osmolality, urine sodium, and urine osmolality to help determine the type and cause of hyponatremia (Cohen and Ellison 2015). For example, low plasma osmolality with high urine osmolality and urine sodium level would be consistent with SIADH, whereas low plasma osmolality with low urine osmolality and urine sodium level would suggest primary polydipsia (Cohen and Ellison 2015). Adrenal insufficiency and severe hypothyroidism can cause hyponatremia, so measuring plasma cortisol and thyroid-stimulating hormone levels may be indicated (Cohen and Ellison 2015). Urine specific gravity and diurnal body weight may be used to monitor psychogenic polydipsia (Iftene et al. 2013).

Management

Hyponatremia, especially when severe, can cause coma, seizures, brain herniation, respiratory arrest, and death (Verbalis et al. 2013). Thus, a patient with severe hyponatremia (as indicated by sodium concentration <120 mEq/L or significant neurological symptoms) will need inpatient medical care and possibly intensive care. Treatment options include fluid restriction and electrolyte replacement with hypertonic (3%) saline; there is mixed evidence regarding the value of replacement with oral sodium tablets and of diuresis with furosemide (Pinkhasov et al. 2021). However, correcting hyponatremia too rapidly also can be dangerous, resulting in brain damage due to osmotic demyelination syndrome (Verbalis et al. 2013). Consultation with a nephrologist or critical care intensivist is recommended for management of severe hyponatremia (Pinkhasov et al. 2021).

For medication-induced SIADH, an important early step is stopping the offending medication (Jacob and Spinler 2006). The risk of discontinuation syndrome (especially with antidepressants) and the need to find an alternative treatment for the underlying psychiatric condition may complicate this. Patients should restrict fluids to approximately 1–1.5 L/day until sodium concentration normalizes, although this recommendation can be difficult to follow; this restriction includes *all* fluid intake, not just water (Jacob and Spinler 2006; Verbalis et al. 2013). Consuming sports drinks may exacerbate hyponatremia because their concentration of electrolytes is minimal (Verbalis et al. 2013). The amount of sodium in the diet should be maintained or, if not contraindicated, increased (Verbalis et al. 2013).

For psychogenic polydipsia, the mainstay of treatment is fluid restriction. If the patient is taking an antipsychotic, switching to clozapine should be considered because some evidence indicates that it may reduce polydipsia (Verbalis et al. 2013). A small uncontrolled trial of group psychotherapy among inpatients with schizophrenia resulted in less polydipsia, but the effect did not persist after the end of therapy (Millson et al. 1993). There are case reports of demeclocycline helping to reduce polydipsia, but a small placebo-controlled trial did not show efficacy (Alexander et al. 1991), and it can cause nephrotoxicity (Pinkhasov et al. 2021).

Follow-Up Management

There is some dilemma as to how best to treat the underlying psychiatric condition in patients with medication-induced hyponatremia. The authors of an expert consensus statement from the Association of Medicine and Psychiatry recommended against rechallenge with the same medication because the risk of developing hyponatremia again is high (Pinkhasov et al. 2021). For patients with depression or an anxiety disorder, switching from one SSRI to another also may result in hyponatremia, although this strategy is reasonable the first time SSRI-induced hyponatremia occurs. Switching from an SSRI to an SNRI is also reasonable, but SNRIs also may cause hyponatremia. The safest antidepressant with respect to hyponatremia is likely bupropion, with mirtazapine being the next safest. Unfortunately, bupropion may not be an effective treatment for anxiety disorders. Whatever alternative antidepressant is prescribed, I recommend close monitoring of sodium concentration. If no antidepressant is tolerable, then psychotherapy and other evidence-based nonpharmacological interventions are indicated. For patients with bipolar disorder who develop hyponatremia with carbamazepine or oxcarbazepine, I recommend switching to another antiepileptic drug or to an antipsychotic medication, with close monitoring of sodium concentration. For patients with hyponatremia at baseline, I recommend prescribing a medication unlikely to exacerbate hyponatremia or using an evidence-based non-pharmacological approach.

Conclusion

Hyponatremia is a common complication of treatment with psychotropic medications, especially in older adults; in those taking thiazide diuretics; and in those with heart failure, liver disease, renal disease, or psychogenic polydipsia. In patients at risk for hyponatremia, clinicians should check sodium concentration prior to starting treatment with an antidepressant, antiepileptic drug (especially carbamazepine and oxcarbazepine), or antipsychotic and then monitor sodium concentration during treatment, especially initially and with titration. Clinicians should maintain a high index of suspicion for hyponatremia in patients who develop confusion or gait instability.

Key Points

Antidepressants, antiepileptic drugs (especially carbamazepine and oxcarbazepine), and antipsychotics have been associated with hyponatremia. Risk factors include older age, female sex, and use of a diuretic medication.

When prescribing an antidepressant, carbamazepine, or oxcarbazepine, I recommend checking the baseline sodium level in patients at risk for developing hyponatremia. I recommend checking again 2 weeks after starting the medication and 2 weeks after each dose increase. If hyponatremia develops, the medication should be stopped.

If a patient taking a psychotropic medication experiences confusion or gait instability, hyponatremia should be considered as a cause.

Treating depression in patients who have had hyponatremia due to antidepressants can be challenging. I recommend considering bupropion, perhaps mirtazapine, psychotherapy, and other evidence-based nonpharmacological treatments.

Psychogenic polydipsia should be considered in patients with severe mental illness who develop hyponatremia.

References

2019 American Geriatrics Society Beers Criteria® Update Expert Panel: American Geriatrics Society 2019 updated AGS Beers Criteria® for Potentially Inappropriate Medication Use in Older Adults. J Am Geriatr Soc 67(4):674–694, 2019 30693946

Alexander RC, Karp BI, Thompson S, et al: A double blind, placebo-controlled trial of demeclocycline treatment of polydipsia-hyponatremia in chronically psychotic patients. Biol Psychiatry 30(4):417–420, 1991 1912134

Berghuis B, Hulst J, Sonsma A, et al: Symptomatology of carbamazepine- and oxcarbazepine-induced hyponatremia in people with epilepsy. Epilepsia 62(3):778–784, 2021 33576502

Cohen DM, Ellison DH: Evaluating hyponatremia. JAMA 313(12):1260–1261, 2015 25803349

De Picker L, Van Den Eede F, Dumont G, et al: Antidepressants and the risk of hyponatremia: a class-by-class review of literature. Psychosomatics 55(6):536–547, 2014 25262043

Fabian TJ, Amico JA, Kroboth PD, et al: Paroxetine-induced hyponatremia in older adults: a 12-week prospective study. Arch Intern Med 164(3):327–332, 2004 14769630

Gandhi S, McArthur E, Mamdani MM, et al: Antiepileptic drugs and hyponatremia in older adults: two population-based cohort studies. Epilepsia 57(12):2067–2079, 2016a 27896804

Gandhi S, McArthur E, Reiss JP, et al: Atypical antipsychotic medications and hyponatremia in older adults: a population-based cohort study. Can J Kidney Health Dis 3:21, 2016b 27069639

Gandhi S, Shariff SZ, Al-Jaishi A, et al: Second-generation antidepressants and hyponatremia risk: a population-based cohort study of older adults. Am J Kidney Dis 69(1):87–96, 2017 27773479

Iftene F, Bowie C, Milev R, et al: Identification of primary polydipsia in a severe and persistent mental illness outpatient population: a prospective observational study. Psychiatry Res 210(3):679–683, 2013 23810384

Illowsky BP, Kirch DG: Polydipsia and hyponatremia in psychiatric patients. Am J Psychiatry 145(6):675–683, 1988 3285701

Jacob S, Spinler SA: Hyponatremia associated with selective serotonin-reuptake inhibitors in older adults. Ann Pharmacother 40(9):1618–1622, 2006 16896026

Liamis G, Milionis H, Elisaf M: A review of drug-induced hyponatremia. Am J Kidney Dis 52(1):144–153, 2008 18468754

Millson RC, Smith AP, Koczapski AB, et al: Self-induced water intoxication treated with group psychotherapy. Am J Psychiatry 150(5):825–826, 1993 8480834

Pinkhasov A, Xiong G, Bourgeois JA, et al: Management of SIADH-related hyponatremia due to psychotropic medications - an expert consensus from the Association of Medicine and Psychiatry. J Psychosom Res 151:110654, 2021 34739943

Ramírez E, Rodríguez A, Queiruga J, et al: Severe hyponatremia is often drug induced: 10-year results of a prospective pharmacovigilance program. Clin Pharmacol Ther 106(6):1362–1379, 2019 31247118

Sailer CO, Winzeler B, Nigro N, et al: Characteristics and outcomes of patients with profound hyponatraemia due to primary polydipsia. Clin Endocrinol (Oxf) 87(5):492–499, 2017 28556237

Shakibaei F, Gholamrezaei A, Alikhani M, Talaeizadeh K: Serum sodium changes in fluoxetine users at different age groups. Iran J Psychiatry 5(3):113–116, 2010 22952503

Verbalis JG, Goldsmith SR, Greenberg A, et al: Diagnosis, evaluation, and treatment of hyponatremia: expert panel recommendations. Am J Med 126(10 Suppl 1):S1–S42, 2013 24074529

Yang H-J, Cheng W-J: Antipsychotic use is a risk factor for hyponatremia in patients with schizophrenia: a 15-year follow-up study. Psychopharmacology (Berl) 234(5):869–876, 2017 28078393

Chapter 10

Neuroleptic Malignant Syndrome

Michael Maksimowski, M.D.

Neuroleptic malignant syndrome (NMS) is a life-threatening medical emergency that was originally discovered in 1960 and termed *syndrome malin des neuroleptiques* after several cases were identified in France in association with the use of haloperidol. The mechanism of action of NMS remains unclear but likely has to do with dopamine receptor imbalance. Activation of proinflammatory cytokines and tumor necrosis factor from antagonism of dopamine receptors results in free radical production and reduced adenosine triphosphate production, which lead to muscle damage and hyperpyrexia (Oruch et al. 2017). Hypothalamic blockade of dopamine receptors is also proposed to be a cause of hyperpyrexia (Figà-Talamanca et al. 1985). Another proposed mechanism of action is a genetic defect in calcium regulatory enzymes within the automatic sympathetic neurons, leading to sympathoadrenal hyperactivity and malignant hyperthermia (Gurrera 2002). Muscle mitochondrial dysfunction may also occur as a primary skeletal muscle defect or direct toxic effect of the offending drug on the skeletal muscle (Gurrera 2002). Other neurotransmitter systems (GABA, epinephrine, serotonin, acetylcholine) also may be involved in pathogenesis (Spivak et al. 2000).

The overall incidence of NMS has been estimated to be 0.16% (Schneider et al. 2020). Two-thirds of cases will manifest within the first week of medication changes, with almost all remaining cases occurring within 30 days (Caroff and Mann 1993). Risk factors include the use of high-potency first-generation antipsychotics (neuroleptics), abrupt discontinuation of dopaminergic agents, family history of NMS (suggesting a genetic basis), dehydration, dementia with Lewy bodies, concomitant use of lithium, and low serum levels of iron (Patil et al. 2014). Age does not appear to be a risk factor. A nationwide inpatient sample within the United States from 2002 to 2011 placed mortality from NMS at 5.6% (Modi et al. 2016), whereas a more recent systematic review of 683 cases from 2018 to 2020 placed mortality from NMS at 7.6% (Guinart et al. 2021a). Predictors of mortality include older age, acute respiratory failure, acute kidney injury, sepsis, and congestive heart failure. Antipsychotic regimen (oral vs. long-acting injectable, typical vs. atypical, monotherapy vs. polytherapy) has not been shown to affect mortality rate (Guinart et al. 2021b). Mortality and incidence rates have declined since the earliest case reports in the 1960s because of greater syndrome awareness, earlier recognition, and better understanding of effective interventions.

Recognition and Detection

NMS often begins as a collection of several unexplained symptoms: altered mental status (agitated delirium, confusion), followed by muscle rigidity, tremor, and/or high blood pressure. Catatonia (e.g., mutism) and choreiform movements also may be seen early in onset. Signs that often occur later in onset are hyperpyrexia and dysautonomia, the latter of which can include diaphoresis, nausea or vomiting, labile blood pressure, tachycardia, tachypnea, and cardiac arrhythmias. Sialorrhea and dysphagia are common and can be complicated by aspiration pneumonia. Signs and symptoms progress rapidly over 2–3 days. NMS can result in coma and death if not identified and treated appropriately.

Culprit Medications

Most cases of NMS are secondary to antipsychotic use. Despite the increased incidence risk with first-generation compared with second-generation antipsychotics, cases of NMS have been associated with almost every antipsychotic (including clozapine). NMS should be high on the list of differential diagnoses when signs and symptoms are coupled with a history of dose initiation or escalation of an antipsychotic or a switch from one antipsychotic to another of similar or greater potency. NMS should be considered less likely in patients taking antipsychotics during a maintenance period or when a dose is slowly increased from a lower standing dose that the patient was already receiving and tolerating well.

Cases also have been seen with the use of antiemetics (e.g., domperidone, droperidol, metoclopramide, prochlorperazine, promethazine). NMS has been associated with discontinuation of tetracyclic and tricyclic antidepressants (e.g., desipramine, dosulepin), monoamine oxidase inhibitors (e.g., phenelzine), selective serotonin reuptake inhibitors (e.g., citalopram), vesicular monoamine transporter inhibitors (e.g., tetrabenazine), anticholinergics, mood stabilizers (e.g., lithium), and anticonvulsants (e.g., valproic acid) (Oruch et al. 2017). Withdrawal from antiparkinsonian drugs (e.g., levodopa, amantadine, anticholinergics) and baclofen also has been associated with NMS.

Assessment

An international consensus study (Gurrera et al. 2011) defined the following criteria for making a diagnosis of NMS, in order of importance:

1. Exposure to dopamine antagonist or dopamine agonist withdrawal within the past 72 hours
2. Hyperthermia (>100.4°F or >38°C, measured orally on at least two occasions)
3. Muscle rigidity
4. Mental status alteration (reduced or fluctuating level of consciousness)
5. Creatine kinase (CK) elevation (at least four times the upper limit of normal levels)
6. Sympathetic nervous system lability, defined as at least two of the following: blood pressure elevation (systolic or diastolic ≥25% above baseline), blood pressure fluctuation (≥20 mm Hg diastolic change or ≥25 mm Hg systolic change within 24 hours), diaphoresis, and urinary incontinence
7. Negative workup for infectious, toxic, metabolic, or neurological causes
8. Hypermetabolism, defined as heart rate increase ≥25% above baseline and respiratory rate increase ≥50% above baseline

A differential diagnosis should include myxedema crisis (secondary to hypothyroidism), malignant catatonia, encephalitis, toxic encephalopathy, malignant hyperpyrexia, heat-stroke, serotonin syndrome, and status epilepticus. Serotonin syndrome is distinguished by the presence of shivering, hyper-reflexia, myoclonus, gastrointestinal symptoms, and/or ataxia. Malignant hyperpyrexia has symptoms identical to NMS but is often more abrupt in onset and includes a history of anesthetic or depolarizing neuromuscular junction blocker use. Malignant catatonia includes a history of prodromal behavioral symptoms (for weeks) before diagnosis and motor symptoms such as dystonia, waxy flexibility, and stereotypies. Clozapine-induced hyperpyrexia is considered a variant of NMS (Bruno et al. 2015) and typically occurs within the first 4 weeks of treatment.

After the initial clinical evaluation, workup should start with a thorough review of hospital drug administration and discontinuation and a history of drug use (both prescription and nonprescription). No diagnostic test is pathognomonic to NMS. Laboratory analysis helps to strengthen the diagnosis and reduce the possibility of other diagnoses. Initial laboratory tests should include a complete blood cell count to monitor for leukocytosis, a metabolic panel to monitor for metabolic acidosis, a CK level to monitor for rhabdomyolysis, and iron studies to monitor for the effects of rhabdomyolysis. Blood tests in NMS will typically show leukocytosis (10,000–40,000 IU/L), thrombocytosis, a CK level that exceeds 1,000 IU/L (and can be as high as 100,000 IU/L), elevated lactate dehydrogenase, and transaminitis. A low serum iron level is sensitive to NMS in most cases (Lee 1998). It is important to remember that CK levels may not be elevated in the early-onset phase of NMS and, when elevated, can be idiopathic or due to other factors such as intramuscular injections and physical restraints. Additional tests such as thyroid panel, liver function tests, blood cultures, toxicological screening, coagulation studies, cerebrospinal fluid analysis, and urine myoglobin tests may be helpful for ruling in or out other conditions. Imaging, such as CT and MRI, is not diagnostically or clinically useful when NMS is strongly suspected but can be used to rule out structural lesions and autoimmune encephalitis, respectively, as causes of altered mental status.

Management

Patients with suspected NMS should be admitted to a medical intensive care unit because of the need for continuous monitoring of cardiorespiratory stability, maintaining a euvolemic state using intravenous fluids, and inserting nasogastric or endotracheal tubing (if necessary). Immediate discontinuation of the offending agent is the most important treatment in NMS, with the exception being when the precipitant is discontinuation of a particular therapy (e.g., dopamine agonist), in which case it should be reinstituted. Cooling blankets and ice packs to the groin and axillae should be used immediately for hyperpyrexia. Rhabdomyolysis can lead to myoglobinemia, hyperkalemia, hyperphosphatemia, hypercalcemia, and hyperuricemia. Electrolyte imbalances can result in cardiac arrhythmias and arrest. Myoglobinemia leads to myoglobinuria and consequent renal failure.

No clear consensus exists on optimal pharmacological treatment for NMS because all recommendations have come from animal models, case studies, and clinical experience rather than human clinical trials (Reulbach et al. 2007). A recent systematic review did not find robust evidence for when or how to choose pharmacological agents to treat NMS (van Rensburg and Decloedt 2019). Any drugs that are used in the treatment of NMS are for symptomatic relief as opposed to treatment of the syndrome itself. Benzodiazepines such as lorazepam are an effective treatment for agitation and catatonia (1–2 mg every 4–6 hours). Dantrolene is a skeletal muscle relaxant that can treat muscular rigidity and reduce heat production (1–2.5 mg/kg IV up to 10 mg/kg/day). Bromocriptine is a dopamine agonist used to restore dopaminergic tone (from 2.5 mg every 6–8 hours to 5 mg every 4 hours up to 40 mg/day). Amantadine is an alternative to bromocriptine with a similar effect (100 mg every 12 hours). Despite limited evidence of efficacy, these medications are frequently used because of the lack of other proven treatments and the high risk of morbidity and mortality. Little to no evidence of efficacy has been seen with levodopa, apomorphine, carbamazepine, or bupropion. Hypertension can be managed effectively with clonidine or nitroprusside. Heparin should be prescribed to prevent deep vein thrombosis.

Electroconvulsive therapy can be used as an alternative treatment for patients who would otherwise be receiving antipsychotics but can also be used to treat malignant catatonia or parkinsonism. However, no prospective or randomized controlled trials support efficacy in the treatment of NMS. One must consider the urgency of treatment and balance this with any safety concerns and whether the patient is able to consent to ECT.

Follow-Up Management

Prognosis depends in part on early diagnosis and active intervention. Most cases will resolve within 1–3 weeks, but with long-acting antipsychotics such as depot injections, some may take 4 weeks or longer. Most patients will not have any neurological sequelae after a full recovery except when hypoxia or prolonged hyperthermia occurred. Should the patient need reinitiation of treatment with an antipsychotic once NMS has subsided, therapy should still be postponed for at least 2 weeks if possible, and a low-potency antipsychotic should be favored to reduce the risk of recurrence of NMS. Lithium therapy is not recommended because it can increase the risk of relapse (Oruch et al. 2014).

Conclusion

NMS is a life-threatening neurological emergency that should be suspected in any patient with acute loss of dopaminergic transmission (i.e., use of antipsychotic or antiemetic or discontinuation of dopaminergic medication) who presents with at least two of the following features: mental status changes, muscle rigidity, fever, and autonomic dysfunction. The most important steps in treatment include discontinuation of the offending agent and restarting dopaminergic agents that were recently discontinued, followed by intensive medical monitoring and treatment until signs and symptoms subside. Clinicians should be familiar with the common signs and symptoms of NMS and ensure that patients are evaluated appropriately whenever antipsychotics are used as part of treatment.

Key Points

The diagnosis of neuroleptic malignant syndrome (NMS) should be suspected when antipsychotics and antiemetics are prescribed or dopamine agonists are discontinued and when two of the following features are present: mental status changes, muscle rigidity, fever, and autonomic dysfunction.

Diagnostic testing can assist in ruling out other conditions and in evaluation of sequelae of NMS.

Management of NMS must be immediate and is based on clinical severity and diagnostic certainty.

Restarting antipsychotic treatment after resolution of NMS is allowed but should be delayed as long as possible. Antipsychotic medications should be titrated slowly, and low-potency second-generation antipsychotics should be favored.

References

Bruno V, Valiente-Gómez A, Alcoverro O: Clozapine and fever: a case of continued therapy with clozapine. Clin Neuropharmacol 38(4):151–153, 2015 26166236

Caroff SN, Mann SC: Neuroleptic malignant syndrome. Med Clin North Am 77(1):185–202, 1993 8093494

Figà-Talamanca L, Gualandi C, Di Meo L, et al: Hyperthermia after discontinuance of levodopa and bromocriptine therapy: impaired dopamine receptors a possible cause. Neurology 35(2):258–261, 1985 3969217

Guinart D, Misawa F, Rubio JM, et al: A systematic review and pooled, patient-level analysis of predictors of mortality in neuroleptic malignant syndrome. Acta Psychiatr Scand 144(4):329–341, 2021a 34358327

Guinart D, Taipale H, Rubio JM, et al: Risk factors, incidence, and outcomes of neuroleptic malignant syndrome on long-acting injectable vs oral antipsychotics in a nationwide schizophrenia cohort. Schizophr Bull 47(6):1621–1630, 2021b 34013325

Gurrera RJ: Is neuroleptic malignant syndrome a neurogenic form of malignant hyperthermia? Clin Neuropharmacol 25(4):183–193, 2002 12151905

Gurrera RJ, Caroff SN, Cohen A, et al: An international consensus study of neuroleptic malignant syndrome diagnostic criteria using the Delphi method. J Clin Psychiatry 72(9):1222–1228, 2011 21733489

Lee JW: Serum iron in catatonia and neuroleptic malignant syndrome. Biol Psychiatry 44(6):499–507, 1998 9777183

Modi S, Dharaiya D, Schultz L, Varelas P: Neuroleptic malignant syndrome: complications, outcomes, and mortality. Neurocrit Care 24(1):97–103, 2016 26223336

Oruch R, Elderbi MA, Khattab HA, et al: Lithium: a review of pharmacology, clinical uses, and toxicity. Eur J Pharmacol 740:464–473, 2014 24991789

Oruch R, Pryme IF, Engelsen BA, Lund A: Neuroleptic malignant syndrome: an easily overlooked neurologic emergency. Neuropsychiatr Dis Treat 13:161–175, 2017 28144147

Patil BS, Subramanyam AA, Singh SL, Kamath RM: Low serum iron as a possible risk factor for neuroleptic malignant syndrome. Int J Appl Basic Med Res 4(2):117–118, 2014 25143888

Reulbach U, Dütsch C, Biermann T, et al: Managing an effective treatment for neuroleptic malignant syndrome. Crit Care 11(1):R4, 2007 17222339

Schneider M, Regente J, Greiner T, et al: Neuroleptic malignant syndrome: evaluation of drug safety data from the AMSP program during 1993–2015. Eur Arch Psychiatry Clin Neurosci 270(1):23–33, 2020 30506147

Spivak B, Maline DI, Vered Y, et al: Prospective evaluation of circulatory levels of catecholamines and serotonin in neuroleptic malignant syndrome. Acta Psychiatr Scand 102(3):226–230, 2000 11008859

van Rensburg R, Decloedt EH: An approach to the pharmacotherapy of neuroleptic malignant syndrome. Psychopharmacol Bull 49(1):84–91, 2019 30858642

Ocular Side Effects of Psychotropic Medications

Haoxing Chen, M.D.
Richard Balon, M.D.

Ocular manifestations of psychotropic medications can be extremely distressing to patients with mental illness because they affect vision and may be accompanied by pain. Reports of ocular side effects of psychotropic medications are uncommon. Most of the presentations are gathered from individual case reports and case series, which form the basis for guidance of management. No medication has been approved by the FDA for management of these effects. It is important for practitioners to be aware of these manifestations, which range from innocuous to potentially vision threatening. Understanding the relationships between visual symptoms and findings associated with a specific class of psychotropic medications allows the provider to effectively manage patient expectations and properly refer patients to eye specialists for escalation of care. Proper and swift management of ocular symptoms not only will help patients to alleviate their fears and better adhere to psychotropic medications but also will decrease the potential for irreversible ocular damage. In this chapter, we review the ocular side effects of psychotropic medications alphabetically. We also mention the most suspected psychotropic medications, or *culprit medications*, associated with these side effects.

Abnormal Pigmentation of External Ocular Structures

Recognition and Detection

Abnormal pigmentation of external ocular structures is recognized by abnormal and often subtle pigment deposition of the eyelids, cornea, and conjunctiva. Patients may report changes in coloration of the eyelids, conjunctiva, or cornea. Pigment deposition has not been described as being associated with any reportable cases of significant visual impairment.

Culprit Medications

Phenothiazines (e.g., chlorpromazine, thioridazine) at high doses (>2 g/day) are the main culprit medications (Richa and Yazbek 2010).

Assessment

Abnormal pigmentation of external ocular structures is assessed by visual inspection. A magnifying glass or ophthalmoscope can be used.

Management

Pigmentation diminishes or resolves after cessation of medication.

Follow-Up Management

If patients are concerned, they should be referred to ophthalmology or optometry specialists for a routine comprehensive evaluation.

Acute Angle-Closure Glaucoma

Glaucoma describes a group of diseases in which the optic nerve is irreversibly damaged (often with associated visual field loss) because of numerous risk factors, one of which is increased intraocular pressure. Damage to the optic nerve can be assessed by direct visualization of the nerve or ophthalmic testing involving visual field testing or imaging of the optic nerve and retinal nerve fiber layer (using, e.g., a Heidelberg Retina Tomograph). Acute angle-closure glaucoma is of particular concern because of the association with numerous psychotropic medications given that prolonged exposure and inadequate management will eventually lead to irreversible blindness. Acute glaucoma is a true emergency.

Two recognized mechanisms lead to acute angle-closure glaucoma. The first one is pupillary block. Many of the medications that can cause mydriasis and cycloplegia (as noted in the "Mydriasis and Cycloplegia" section) of the pupils via anti-adrenergic and anticholinergic mechanisms can also cause pupillary block. The dilation of pupils causes the iris to rest in a position in relation to the lens that blocks flow of aqueous fluid from the ciliary body to the trabecular meshwork drainage angle in the anterior chamber. This mechanism is more likely to occur in patients who have less space in the anterior chamber in the relationship between the iris and the lens (e.g., hyperopic, or *farsighted*, vision). As the aqueous fluid builds up, the intraocular pressure increases in the eye (Jain et al. 2021). The second mechanism that leads to acute angle-closure glaucoma is nonpupillary block. In this mechanism, the iris does not directly contact the lens to block the flow of aqueous fluid. Alternatively, anterior rotation and swelling of the ciliary body push the peripheral iris forward to oppose and directly block the trabecular meshwork responsible for drainage. Partial or complete blockage will lead to aqueous fluid buildup, resulting in an increase in intraocular pressure (Jain et al. 2021).

Recognition and Detection

The most prominent symptom of acute angle-closure glaucoma is sudden severe eye pain in one or both eyes (medication-associated glaucoma often affects both eyes). Further symptoms include eye redness, mid-dilated pupil, haziness of the cornea, nausea, and vomiting. Patients also complain of sudden blurry and decreased vision, seeing circles around lights, headache, brow pain, eye pain, and extreme sensitivity to light.

Culprit Medications

Pupillary block can theoretically occur with the use of any of the medications that can cause mydriasis and cycloplegia (noted in the "Mydriasis and Cycloplegia" section) but has commonly been associated with tricyclic antidepressants (TCAs) and selective serotonin reuptake inhibitors (SSRIs) (i.e., paroxetine, citalopram, escitalopram, fluoxetine, fluvoxamine). The nonpupillary block mechanism is most commonly associated with topiramate.

Assessment

An ophthalmologist should measure intraocular pressure and perform a gonioscopy to evaluate possible damage. Further glaucoma testing with visual field assessment and scans of the optic nerve or retinal fiber layers can quantify the severity of damage.

Management

The suspected offending agent should be stopped urgently, and the patient should be sent for evaluation of possible damage to the retina and optic nerve.

Follow-Up Management

The patient should be urgently referred to a comprehensive ophthalmologist or glaucoma specialist for a topical or systemic ocular antihypertensive and possible laser or surgical management because persistent elevated intraocular pressure will lead to irreversible vision loss.

Special Note

Patients with a history of glaucoma should be cautiously advised and monitored if any of the culprit medications (e.g., TCAs) are to be recommended. It is prudent for these patients to schedule a routine evaluation with their eye specialist to evaluate risk for acute angle-closure glaucoma prior to starting the medication and to be seen routinely afterward.

Eye Movement Abnormalities Not Associated With Oculogyric Crisis

Various eye movement abnormalities have been observed and are associated with psychotropic agents because of broad effects on the CNS. The mechanism of these movements varies by medication but involves areas of the brain responsible for gaze fixation, saccade (quick reflexive eye movement) generation, and object pursuit.

Recognition and Detection

Eye movement abnormalities are recognized through visible impairment of normal eye movements or new development of abnormal eye movements that are spontaneous or rhythmic. Patients typically complain of intermittent double vision, uncontrolled eye movements, or oscillopsia (the sensation that the viewed image or environment is constantly moving).

Culprit Medications

Benzodiazepines can cause interruption of normal saccadic and smooth-pursuit eye movements with a compromised ability to track moving objects. Lithium can lead to downbeat nystagmus (continuous slow upward movement of eyes followed by a quick downward compensatory movement). Carbamazepine can lead to a decreased ability to converge the eyes, difficulty holding a steady gaze, difficulty tracking objects, and difficulty initiating saccades. Nystagmus (any direction, although usually downbeat) has been noted with high doses of lamotrigine, and nystagmus (any direction) can also occur with high doses of topiramate (Richa and Yazbek 2010).

Assessment

Eye movement abnormalities are assessed through visual inspection and monitoring.

Management

Cessation of the suspected medication usually leads to improvement or resolution of symptoms.

Follow-Up Management

Close monitoring and careful introduction of any new psychotropic medications are advised. Patients with persistent or worsening eye movements should be referred to neuropsychiatry, neurology, or neuro-ophthalmology for further evaluation.

Mydriasis and Cycloplegia

Mydriasis refers to the phenomenon in which the pupil dilates under natural or iatrogenic conditions. Cycloplegia refers to the phenomenon in which the ciliary muscles are compromised, resulting in an inability to accommodate (i.e., focus up close). The systemic anticholinergic effect of various medications on the ciliary body can cause cycloplegia. The anticholinergic effect of various medications on ocular structures can also cause passive dilation of the pupils by inhibiting the para-sympathetic innervation of the iris sphincter muscle. Although the mechanism is not completely clear, mydriasis is caused by sympathomimetic action via interference with reuptake of norepinephrine or increased activation of α_1-adrenergic receptors in the pupillary dilator muscles (Richa and Yazbek 2010).

Recognition and Detection

Mydriasis and cycloplegia cause recognizable increased dilation of the pupils from baseline (usually >6 mm in size) and difficulty reading up close. Patients will complain of blurry vision, increased sensitivity to light, and difficulty reading.

Culprit Medications

Culprit medications include phenothiazines, other antipsychotics, TCAs, SSRIs, and topiramate.

Assessment

Mydriasis and cycloplegia are assessed through visual inspection, pupil measurement, and a reading ability evaluation.

Management

Impaired vision tends to improve with time if medications are continued and often resolves with cessation of suspected medications.

Follow-Up Management

Patients should be monitored carefully over time to ensure that they have no associated significant ocular pain, discomfort, or drastic sustained decrease in vision. If the aforementioned symptoms occur or symptoms persist once the culprit medication is stopped, then urgent referral to an ophthalmologist or optometrist is necessary.

Oculogyric Crisis

Oculogyric crisis is a subclass of a condition called dystonia in which involuntary contraction of various muscles in the body occurs (see Chapter 1, "Acute Dystonia"). Dystonia can be extremely discomforting and painful. Any or all ocular muscles can be involved. Extraocular muscular dystonia is thought to be caused by dopaminergic-cholinergic imbalance from the dopamine receptor blockade of certain psychotropic medications. Case studies have shown that effects are dose independent and can occur even at therapeutic dosages (Slow and Lang 2017).

Recognition and Detection

Sustained involuntary contraction of multiple extraocular muscles leads to decreased or paralyzed eye movements that can last from seconds to hours. The most common presentation is the eyes being fixed in an upward gaze. Patients will complain about painful, uncontrolled eye movements.

Culprit Medications

Butyrophenones, phenothiazines, risperidone, olanzapine, aripiprazole, carbamazepine, topiramate, and escitalopram are described in the literature as being associated with oculogyric crisis.

Assessment

Oculogyric crisis is assessed through visual inspection.

Management

Administration of intramuscular benztropine 1–2 mg, oral diphenhydramine 50 mg, or intramuscular lorazepam 1–2 mg (Richa and Yazbek 2010) relieves acute symptomatology. If possible, culprit medications should be stopped, and patients should be switched to alternatives. Prophylaxis with benztropine can be considered in patients with significant increase in medication dose or a history of dystonic attacks.

Follow-Up Management

Patients should be closely monitored by a neuropsychiatrist and neurologist if attacks are reoccurring and persistent.

Pigmentary Cataract Deposits

Cataract deposits are granular pigment depositions near the anterior capsule of the lens that are detectable only by an ophthalmologist using a slit lamp device.

Recognition and Detection

Commonly, patients have no visual symptoms. Rarely, patients observe mildly progressive blurring of vision after starting the medication.

Culprit Medications

Phenothiazines, especially chlorpromazine and thioridazine (>800 mg/day), are the main culprit medications (Richa and Yazbek 2010).

Assessment

Cataract deposits are found through an ophthalmologic examination (visual) using a slit lamp.

Management

An eye specialist may recommend that the psychiatrist decrease the dose or stop or switch medications if a visually significant cataract starts to develop and patients report blurry or decreased vision. Cataract surgery may be necessary in extreme cases.

Follow-Up Management

Patients should be referred to ophthalmology or optometry specialists for routine comprehensive evaluation and/or further care.

Pigmentary Retinal Deposits

Granular pigment depositions or pigment changes associated with various psychotropic medications may develop in the retina because of high vascularization of this structure.

Recognition and Detection

Patients may complain of blurry vision, decreased peripheral vision, and decreased nighttime vision. Granular pigment depositions or pigment changes are noted in the retina on dilated fundus examination by an ophthalmic specialist. The depositions often start in the periphery and then gradually accumulate toward the center of vision (Li et al. 2008).

Culprit Medications

Phenothiazines, especially chlorpromazine and thioridazine (>800 mg/day), and carbamazepine are the main culprit medications (Richa and Yazbek 2010).

Assessment

Granular pigment depositions are assessed during an ophthalmologic examination via fundoscopy after dilating the pupil.

Management

An eye specialist may recommend that the psychiatrist decrease the dose or stop or switch the medication if retinal findings are apparent and the patient is experiencing visual symptoms.

Follow-Up Management

Patients should be referred to ophthalmology or optometry specialists for routine comprehensive evaluation, including visual field testing.

Visual Disturbances Related to Phosphodiesterase Inhibitors

Psychiatrists may prescribe phosphodiesterase type 5 (PDE5) inhibitors (e.g., sildenafil) for erectile dysfunction associated with various psychotropic medications. All PDE5 inhibitors also weakly inhibit PDE6 located in the rod and cone photoreceptors, which can cause visual changes correlating with plasma levels—namely, blue tinge (Kerr and Danesh-Meyer 2009; Moschos and Nitoda 2016).

Recognition and Detection

Patients may complain of blurry vision and bluish tinge in vision, especially when focusing on objects with darker shades of color, and changes in light perception (in 6%–18% of men taking sildenafil).

Culprit Medications

PDE5 inhibitors (avanafil, sildenafil, tadalafil, vardenafil) are the main culprit medications. Symptoms are dose dependent.

Assessment

Visual disturbances related to phosphodiesterase inhibitors are assessed through patient reporting or active questioning.

Management

Symptoms are often temporary and should be monitored closely. No definitive studies have found permanent toxic effects of phosphodiesterase inhibitors on the ocular structures. Patients should be educated about this benign side effect.

Follow-Up Management

Patients should be referred to ophthalmology or optometry specialists for routine comprehensive evaluation if visual symptoms persist.

Conclusion

Ocular side effects are relatively infrequent but can be distressing to patients and can potentially cause severe damage. Some of them—namely, acute angle-closure glaucoma and oculogyric crisis—are true emergencies. Patients with ocular side effects should be referred to an ophthalmologist (acute glaucoma) in some cases but can be managed by psychiatrists (oculogyric crisis) in other cases. A careful history (e.g., of preexisting glaucoma) and astute observation combined with good listening skills regarding patients' reports of symptoms help to establish the diagnosis in most cases. For certain preexisting conditions, careful monitoring is necessary (e.g., TCA use with preexisting glaucoma). Psychiatrists' involvement in the management of ocular side effects should include psychoeducation (explanation of side effects), medication cessation or modification, and collaboration with an ophthalmologist.

Key Points

Ocular side effects can be emergent and cause ocular damage.

It is essential for psychiatrists to gather a careful history related to ocular symptoms.

Psychiatrist involvement in the management of ocular side effects includes psychoeducation, discontinuation or change of medication, and close collaboration with ophthalmologists.

Recommended Readings

Li J, Tripathi RC, Tripathi BJ: Drug-induced ocular disorders. Drug Saf 31(2):127–141, 2008 18217789

Richa S, Yazbek JC: Ocular adverse effects of common psychotropic agents: a review. CNS Drugs 24(6):501–526, 2010 20443647

References

Jain NS, Ruan CW, Dhanji SR, Symes RJ: Psychotropic drug-induced glaucoma: a practical guide to diagnosis and management. CNS Drugs 35(3):283–289, 2021 33604881

Kerr NM, Danesh-Meyer HV: Phosphodiesterase inhibitors and the eye. Clin Exp Ophthalmol 37(5):514–523, 2009 19624350

Li J, Tripathi RC, Tripathi BJ: Drug-induced ocular disorders. Drug Saf 31(2):127–141, 2008 18217789

Moschos MM, Nitoda E: Pathophysiology of visual disorders induced by phosphodiesterase inhibitors in the treatment of erectile dysfunction. Drug Des Devel Ther 8:3407–3413, 2016 27799745

Richa S, Yazbek JC: Ocular adverse effects of common psychotropic agents: a review. CNS Drugs 24(6):501–526, 2010 20443647

Slow EJ, Lang AE: Oculogyric crises: a review of phenomenology, etiology, pathogenesis, and treatment. Mov Disord 32(2):193–202, 2017 28218460

Overdoses of Psychotropic Medications

Antidepressants, Lithium, and Antipsychotics

Spencer Greene, M.D., M.S., FACEP,
FACMT, FAACT, FAAEM

Antidepressants and other psychotropic medications are among the most frequently prescribed drugs in the United States, and adverse effects are commonly reported to U.S. poison centers. Toxicity may be idiosyncratic, result from acute overdose, or develop following chronic use. In 2019, there were 137,881 calls to U.S. poison centers involving antidepressants and 135,091 concerning antipsychotics (Gummin et al. 2020). No class of drugs is implicated in more fatal ingestions than antipsychotics, and the various types of antidepressants are collectively ranked second for fatal ingestions in patients older than 20 years. Furthermore, the number of cases involving antidepressants rose more than for any other class of drugs between 2018 and 2019.

Lithium is much less commonly prescribed than it previously was and than other medications because it has been replaced by newer medications, such as valproic acid, carbamazepine, and antipsychotics, that have better safety profiles. In 2019, poison centers were contacted for 7,085 cases, including 4 fatalities and an additional 197 patients who had potentially life-threatening signs and symptoms (Gummin et al. 2020).

Antidepressants

Tricyclic Antidepressants

Recognition and Detection

Tricyclic antidepressants (TCAs) provide their therapeutic effect by increasing concentrations of serotonin and norepinephrine. Some of the toxicities observed in overdose can be directly attributed to excessive activity of these neurotransmitters. Excessive norepinephrine can result in hypertension and tachycardia. Serotonergic features include altered mental status, tachycardia, mydriasis, labile blood pressure, clonus, hyperreflexia, hyperthermia, tremor, and rigidity, particularly in the lower extremities. Patients may have significant toxicity without satisfying the formal criteria for serotonin syndrome (Boyer and Shannon 2005).

Serotonin toxicity can also occur idiosyncratically in therapeutic use. Signs and symptoms appear within 24 hours of starting or increasing the dose of a serotonergic medication. Toxicity is particularly likely if the serotonergic medications have mechanisms that work additively or synergistically.

Other clinical features of TCA toxicity are unrelated to their primary mechanism(s) of action. Inhibition of sodium channels leads to a delayed action potential, resulting in hypotension and QRS complex widening on an electrocardiogram (ECG). Blockade of potassium efflux leads to QT interval prolongation on an ECG. Muscarinic antagonism produces an antimuscarinic toxidrome, characterized by tachycardia, mydriasis, mumbling speech, ileus, anhidrosis, urinary retention, and altered mental status that can range from CNS depression to delirium. Antagonism of peripheral α_1-adrenergic receptors causes vasodilation, resulting in hypotension and reflex tachycardia. Miosis also may result from this adrenergic antagonism. Seizures result from antagonism of GABA receptors (Greene et al. 2017).

Because TCAs exert toxicity via multiple and occasionally competing mechanisms, clinical features may vary. Tachycardia, hypotension, altered mental status, and ECG abnormalities are most consistently seen and appear within 4 hours of ingestion. Seizures are common in overdoses of greater than 10 mg/kg. The skin is warm but may be moist or dry. Similarly, pupil size and bowel activity are unpredictable.

Assessment

Laboratory tests and an ECG should be obtained for all symptomatic patients and following intentional ingestions (Nazarian et al. 2017). Measuring acetaminophen and salicylate levels is recommended to exclude coingestion. Although semiquantitative TCA level tests are available in some hospitals, the results rarely affect management. Because the therapeutic range is so wide, a level that may indicate toxicity in one patient may be subtherapeutic in another individual.

Other recommended blood tests include a complete blood count, basic metabolic profile, and ethanol level. A pregnancy test should be obtained for postmenarchal, premenopausal women. Additional tests should be performed as clinically indicated.

Mental health professionals commonly request a urine drug screen, particularly when inpatient hospitalization is being considered. The limitation of these tests must be recognized (Eisen et al. 2004). Only specific drugs and drug classes are included; the vast majority of potential ingestants can go undetected. Furthermore, false-positive and false-negative results are common. As a result, some patients receive unnecessary testing and treatment, whereas others go without necessary treatment. This is especially true for TCAs because more than a dozen medications can produce a false-positive TCA result.

Management

Management of TCA toxicity is primarily supportive. A patent airway should be established, and adequate oxygenation and ventilation should be ensured. Euvolemia should be maintained. Hypotension that fails to respond to fluid resuscitation with crystalloid solutions should be treated with direct-acting vasopressors such as norepinephrine. Sodium bicarbonate boluses are recommended for QRS complex widening (Bradberry et al. 2005). Magnesium sulfate should be administered intravenously for QT interval prolongation, and potassium should be supplemented as needed to maintain a level greater than 4.0 mEq/L.

Toxicity-induced seizures are best treated with benzodiazepines or other direct-acting GABA agonists. Phenytoin and levetiracetam are typically ineffective.

Benzodiazepines are first-line pharmacotherapy for serotonin toxicity. Cyproheptadine, a serotonergic histamine antagonist, is indicated for refractory serotonin toxicity but works slowly and must be given enterally.

Physostigmine should be considered for antimuscarinic delirium. There is a misconception that physostigmine is contraindicated in TCA toxicity. In fact, it is safe and effective in the absence of actual contraindications, which include allergy to any component of the drug, severe asthma, bradycardia, atrioventricular block, and mechanical obstruction of the gastrointestinal (GI) or genitourinary tract (Suchard 2003). If physostigmine is unavailable, other centrally acting cholinesterase inhibitors, such as rivastigmine, may be used.

Because TCAs are absorbed rapidly, gastrointestinal decontamination (GID) is unlikely to be effective (Greene et al. 2008). Furthermore, if CNS depression occurs, GID may significantly increase the risk of pulmonary aspiration of gastric contents.

Follow-Up Management

Patients who intentionally overdose require psychiatric consultation once they are medically stabilized. Patients with idiosyncratic serotonin toxicity should have their medications adjusted, which may include discontinuation of one or more serotonergic medications.

Selective Serotonin Reuptake Inhibitors

Recognition and Detection

Selective serotonin reuptake inhibitors (SSRIs) increase serotonin levels, which can lead to serotonin toxicity in overdose or idiopathically. Acute SSRI overdoses most commonly cause CNS depression, GI symptoms, and tachycardia. Seizures and ECG abnormalities, including QRS complex widening and QT interval prolongation, may be observed, particularly following citalopram or, to a lesser extent, escitalopram ingestions (Engebretsen et al. 2003; Klein-Schwartz et al. 2012).

Assessment

As mentioned in the previous "Tricyclic Antidepressants" subsection, laboratory tests, including acetaminophen and salicylate levels, and an ECG should be obtained for all symptomatic patients and following intentional ingestions. Patients should be monitored for at least 8 hours from time of ingestion.

Management

A patent airway, adequate oxygenation and ventilation, and euvolemia should be ensured; benzodiazepines are recommended for seizures and serotonergic toxicity. Sodium bicarbonate boluses should be used for QRS complex widening, whereas QT interval prolongation is treated with magnesium sulfate supplementation and potassium optimization.

Follow-Up Management

Intentional overdoses require psychiatric evaluation. Patients with idiosyncratic serotonin toxicity should have their medications adjusted, which may include discontinuation of one or more serotonergic medications.

Serotonin-Norepinephrine Reuptake Inhibitors

Recognition and Detection

Serotonin-norepinephrine reuptake inhibitors (SNRIs) increase serotonin and norepinephrine levels. Acute SNRI overdoses most commonly cause CNS depression, GI symptoms, hypertension, and tachycardia. Seizures and ECG abnormalities, including QRS complex widening and QT interval prolongation, may be observed. Because venlafaxine comes as an extended-release (ER) product, signs and symptoms may be delayed.

Assessment

Laboratory tests, including acetaminophen and salicylate levels, and an ECG should be obtained for all symptomatic patients and following intentional ingestions. Patients with venlafaxine ER ingestions should be monitored for at least 12 hours because of the potential for delayed toxicity.

Management

A patent airway, adequate oxygenation and ventilation, and euvolemia should be ensured. Benzodiazepines are recommended for seizures and serotonergic toxicity. Sodium bicarbonate boluses should be used for QRS complex widening, whereas QT interval prolongation is treated with magnesium sulfate supplementation and potassium optimization. Single-dose activated charcoal 1 g/kg is a reasonable way to perform

GID in asymptomatic, cooperative patients with venlafaxine ER ingestions without other contraindications.

Follow-Up Management

Intentional overdoses require psychiatric evaluation. Patients with idiosyncratic serotonin toxicity should have their medications adjusted, which may include discontinuation of one or more serotonergic medications.

Miscellaneous Antidepressants

Recognition and Detection

Although trazodone is both a serotonin agonist and a reuptake inhibitor, serotonin toxicity is not typically observed in overdose. Toxicity is generally limited to CNS depression, although bradycardia and, occasionally, QT interval prolongation may be observed.

Mirtazapine antagonizes central α_2-adrenergic receptors and histamine receptors. Toxicity manifests as CNS depression. Serotonin toxicity is not observed.

Bupropion, which inhibits the reuptake of norepinephrine and dopamine, is especially dangerous in overdose. Through mechanisms that have yet to be fully elucidated, bupropion also causes seizures and QRS and QT interval abnormalities (Caillier et al. 2012). Toxicity is delayed following ingestions of sustained-release (SR) or ER products. Serotonin toxicity has been described following bupropion overdoses, although this is controversial.

Assessment

Laboratory tests, including acetaminophen and salicylate levels, and an ECG should be obtained for all symptomatic patients and following intentional ingestions. Patients with bupropion SR and ER ingestions should be monitored for at least 24 hours because of the potential for delayed toxicity.

Management

A patent airway, adequate oxygenation and ventilation, and euvolemia should be ensured. Benzodiazepines are recommended for seizures and serotonergic toxicity. Sodium bicarbonate boluses should be used for QRS complex widening, whereas QT interval prolongation is treated with magnesium sulfate supplementation and potassium optimization. Note that bupropion-induced ECG abnormalities often fail to respond to standard therapy. Single-dose activated charcoal 1 g/kg should be considered for asymptomatic, cooperative patients with bupropion SR or ER ingestions without other contraindications.

Follow-Up Management

Intentional overdoses require psychiatric evaluation. Patients with idiosyncratic serotonin toxicity should have their medications adjusted, which may include discontinuation of one or more serotonergic medications.

Lithium

Recognition and Detection

Acute lithium overdoses directly irritate the GI tract, leading to vomiting and diarrhea. Volume loss can be significant. Neurological findings may develop over time if patients go untreated. Chronic toxicity develops in patients who have been taking a stable dose for more than 1–2 weeks when the dose is excessive or when an acute decrease in renal elimination occurs, such as in the setting of acute volume loss from concomitant use of angiotensin converting enzyme inhibitors or nonsteroidal anti-inflammatory drugs. It is characterized primarily by neurological toxicity, which may include tremor, clonus, hyperreflexia, nystagmus, dysarthria, ataxia, encephalopathy, and seizure (Okusa and Crystal 1994). The syndrome of irreversible lithium-effectuated neurotoxicity (SILENT) develops in a fraction of these patients. Nonneurological sequelae may include nephrogenic diabetes insipidus, hyperparathyroidism, and hypothyroidism. Acute-on-chronic toxicity manifests with mild to moderate GI symptoms followed shortly by neurological toxicity. Endocrine and renal dysfunction also may be present.

Assessment

In addition to laboratory testing for acetaminophen and salicylate coingestion and an ECG, serial lithium levels should be measured until a downward trend is clear. In acute toxicity, the lithium level may be significantly elevated in patients without neurological symptoms because the drug has not distributed into the brain. Conversely, patients with chronic toxicity may present with severe symptoms despite modestly elevated levels. It is essential to use the correct blood tube to measure lithium levels because certain tubes already contain lithium (in the form of lithium heparin), which will result in a spurious reading. Because renal insufficiency may contribute to chronic lithium toxicity, serum urea nitrogen and serum creatinine levels may be elevated. Hypercalcemia and thyroid abnormalities also may be present. Serum levels of carbamazepine and valproic acid should be measured in patients with bipolar disorder who also may be prescribed these medications.

Management

Lithium carbonate is an ER formulation and is therefore amenable to GID. However, lithium is not adsorbable by single-dose activated charcoal. For awake, cooperative patients with acute or acute-on-chronic lithium overdoses, whole bowel irrigation using high-molecular-weight polyethylene glycol electrolyte solution should be performed.

A patent airway, adequate oxygenation and ventilation, and euvolemia should be ensured. Normal saline is preferable because sodium can enhance lithium excretion. Benzodiazepines are recommended for seizures and serotonergic toxicity. Lithium is a small, polar, water-soluble compound with minimal protein binding, so hemodialysis should be considered when patients with chronic lithium toxicity are encephalopathic, have had a seizure, or have renal insufficiency (Jaeger et al. 1993).

Follow-Up Management

Patients who intentionally overdose require psychiatric consultation once they are medically stabilized. Patients with idiosyncratic serotonin toxicity should have their medications adjusted, which may include discontinuation of one or more serotonergic medications. In cases of chronic lithium toxicity, it is essential to determine whether the dose was chronically elevated, a transient decrease in renal function was caused by volume depletion, or renal function was impaired by concomitant medication use.

Antipsychotics

Typical Antipsychotics

Recognition and Detection

Antipsychotics, also referred to as neuroleptics, have several mechanisms of action, the most significant of which is antagonism of 70%–80% of dopamine D_2 receptors. Low-potency typical antipsychotics such as chlorpromazine cause CNS depression and antimuscarinic toxicity in overdose. However, because of the peripheral α_1-adrenergic receptor blockade, miosis, rather than mydriasis, is common. Adrenergic antagonism also causes hypotension and tachycardia. QRS complex widening, QT interval prolongation, and seizures may be observed. High-potency butyrophenone antipsychotics, such as haloperidol and droperidol, may cause CNS depression, seizures, and QT interval prolongation in overdose.

Extrapyramidal side effects (EPS) may develop during therapeutic neuroleptic use, particularly with butyrophenones and risperidone. Several presentations are possible, including dystonia, akathisia, parkinsonism, and tardive dyskinesia. Neuroleptic malignant syndrome (NMS) is sometimes considered an extreme form of EPS. Most cases develop within the first week, but up to 10% of NMS cases will appear weeks to months after starting an antipsychotic. NMS has many of the clinical features of serotonin syndrome. They are both characterized by altered mental status, tachycardia, labile blood pressure, and hyperthermia (Caroff and Mann 1993). Clonus, tremor, and shivering are more suggestive of serotonin syndrome. Bradykinesia is observed with NMS. The rigidity seen in NMS typically affects the upper extremities and is commonly described as *lead pipe* (Gurrera et al. 2011). The rigidity of serotonin syndrome is usually confined to the lower extremities and is not as profound.

Assessment

ECG and laboratory tests, including acetaminophen and salicylate levels, are recommended for assessment.

Management

Treatment is supportive, with an emphasis on airway, breathing, and circulation. Hypotension that fails to respond to fluid resuscitation with crystalloid solutions should be treated with direct-acting vasopressors such as norepinephrine. Sodium bicarbonate boluses are recommended for QRS complex widening. Magnesium sulfate should be administered intravenously for QT interval prolongation, and potassium should be supplemented as needed to maintain a level greater than 4.0 mEq/L.

Toxicity-induced seizures are best treated with benzodiazepines or other direct-acting GABA agonists. Phenytoin and levetiracetam are typically ineffective.

Physostigmine should be considered for antimuscarinic delirium. If physostigmine is unavailable, other centrally acting cholinesterase inhibitors, such as rivastigmine, may be used.

Typical antipsychotics are absorbed rapidly, so GID is unlikely to be effective. Because these medications are also lipophilic and highly protein bound, hemodialysis is ineffective and therefore is not recommended.

Antimuscarinic drugs, such as benztropine and diphenhydramine, are indicated for dystonia. β-Adrenergic receptor antagonists and benzodiazepines are recommended for akathisia. Benzodiazepines are also the recommended initial pharmacotherapy for NMS. The dopamine analogue bromocriptine should be used to treat NMS that fails to improve with benzodiazepines. Bromocriptine works slowly and must be given enterally. Dantrolene, which works peripherally, is not the antidote for NMS. It may be used to reduce rigidity, but because it lacks CNS effects, it cannot be used as monotherapy.

Follow-Up Management

Patients who intentionally overdose require psychiatric consultation once they are medically stabilized. Patients with EPS or NMS should have their medications reviewed and adjusted as needed after consideration of risks, benefits, and alternatives.

Atypical Antipsychotics

Recognition and Detection

Atypical antipsychotics antagonize 40%–60% of D_2 receptors and also antagonize 70%–90% of serotonin type 2A (5-HT_{2A}) receptors. Clinical features of benzepine atypical antipsychotic (e.g., clozapine, olanzapine, quetiapine) overdoses resemble acute toxicity from low-potency typical neuroleptics. Quetiapine is particularly sedating, whereas olanzapine is the most antimuscarinic. Because clozapine is an agonist at the muscarinic M_4 receptor, sialorrhea, rather than dry mouth, is present. Chronic benzepine toxicity includes weight gain, hyperglycemia, and—with clozapine—agranulocytosis and myocarditis.

Acute overdoses of indole antipsychotics (e.g., risperidone, paliperidone, ziprasidone, lurasidone) result in CNS depression, hypotension, tachycardia, and miosis. QRS complex widening is not observed, but QT interval prolongation may develop, especially with the use of ziprasidone. Seizure is possible, particularly with the use of risperidone. Toxicity from quinolinones such as aripiprazole is limited to CNS depression and, occasionally, hypotension.

Assessment

ECG and laboratory tests, including acetaminophen and salicylate levels, are recommended for assessment. Patients with paliperidone ingestions should be monitored for at least 24 hours because of the potential for delayed toxicity.

Management

Treatment is supportive, with an emphasis on airway, breathing, and circulation. Hypotension that fails to respond to fluid resuscitation with crystalloid solutions should be treated with direct-acting vasopressors such as norepinephrine. Sodium bicarbonate boluses are recommended for QRS complex widening. Magnesium sulfate should be administered intravenously for QT interval prolongation, and potassium should be supplemented as needed to maintain a level greater than 4.0 mEq/L.

Toxicity-induced seizures are best treated with benzodiazepines or other direct-acting GABA agonists. Physostigmine should be considered for antimuscarinic delirium. If physostigmine is unavailable, other centrally acting cholinesterase inhibitors, such as rivastigmine, may be used. Because paliperidone has delayed and prolonged absorption, GID with single-dose activated charcoal should be performed in asymptomatic, cooperative patients with no other contraindications.

Follow-Up Management

Patients who intentionally overdose require psychiatric consultation once they are medically stabilized. Patients with

EPS or NMS should have their medications reviewed and adjusted as needed after consideration of risks, benefits, and alternatives. Patients taking clozapine need to have their blood counts monitored. Cardiology consultation is recommended for patients with suspected cardiomyopathy, and endocrinology referrals should be arranged for patients who have hyperglycemia.

Conclusion

Toxicity from psychotropic medications, whether it is caused by acute overdose, chronic use, or idiosyncratic reactions, is not uncommon. Neurological effects are most often observed and may include CNS depression, delirium, and encephalopathy. Hypotension and electrocardiographic manifestations such as QRS complex widening and QT interval prolongation may be observed. Many antidepressants and lithium can cause serotonergic toxicity. Acute overdoses of TCAs, low-potency typical antipsychotics, and benzepine antipsychotics may produce an antimuscarinic toxidrome. EPS can be observed in therapeutic use of many neuroleptics, particularly high-potency typical antipsychotics and risperidone. Treatment for these various manifestations is primarily supportive. In select cases, antidotal therapy may be warranted, and consultation with the regional poison control center is recommended.

Key Points

The most clinically significant features of antidepressant overdose include hypotension, tachycardia, seizures, electrocardiographic abnormalities, and serotonergic toxicity.

Acute lithium toxicity initially manifests as gastrointestinal symptoms. Neurological toxicity, which is the hallmark of chronic lithium toxicity, develops only in patients who go untreated.

Acute antipsychotic toxicity is characterized by CNS depression and occasionally hypotension. Select drugs may cause cardiotoxicity, seizures, and an antimuscarinic toxidrome.

The mainstay of treatment for psychotropic medication overdoses is supportive care.

Benzodiazepines are the first-line treatment for serotonin toxicity, neuroleptic malignant syndrome, and drug-induced seizures.

Centrally acting cholinesterase inhibitors, such as physostigmine, can treat antimuscarinic toxicity.

QRS complex widening is best treated with sodium bicarbonate, whereas QT interval prolongation is corrected with magnesium supplementation and potassium optimization.

References

Boyer EW, Shannon M: The serotonin syndrome. N Engl J Med 352(11):1112–1120, 2005 15784664

Bradberry SM, Thanacoody HK, Watt BE, et al: Management of the cardiovascular complications of tricyclic antidepressant poisoning: role of sodium bicarbonate. Toxic Rev 24(3):195–204, 2005 16390221

Caillier B, Pilote S, Castonguay A, et al: QRS and QT prolongation under bupropion: a unique cardiac electrophysiological profile. Fundam Clin Pharmacol 26(5):599–608, 2012 21623902

Caroff SN, Mann SC: Neuroleptic malignant syndrome. Med Clin North Am 77(1):185–202, 1993 8093494

Eisen JS, Sivilotti ML, Boyd KU, et al: Screening urine for drugs of abuse in the emergency department: do test results affect physicians' patient care decisions? CJEM 6(2):104–111, 2004 17433159

Engebretsen KM, Harris CR, Wood JE: Cardiotoxicity and late onset seizures with citalopram overdose. J Emerg Med 25(2):163–166, 2003 12902002

Greene S, Harris C, Singer J: Gastrointestinal decontamination of the poisoned patient. Pediatr Emerg Care 24(3):176–186, 2008 18347499

Greene S, AufderHeide E, French-Rojas L: Toxicological emergencies in patients with mental illness: when medications are no longer your friends. Psychiatr Clin North Am 40(3):519–532, 2017 28800806

Gummin DD, Mowry JB, Beuhler MC, et al: 2019 annual report of the American Association of Poison Control Centers' National Poison Data System (NPDS): 37th annual report. Clin Toxicol (Phila) 58(12):1360–1541, 2020 33305966

Gurrera RJ, Caroff SN, Cohen A, et al: An international consensus study of neuroleptic malignant syndrome diagnostic criteria using the Delphi method. J Clin Psychiatry 72(9):1222–1228, 2011 21733489

Jaeger A, Sauder P, Kopferschmitt J, et al: When should dialysis be performed in lithium poisoning? A kinetic study in 14 cases of lithium poisoning. J Toxicol Clin Toxicol 31(3):429–447, 1993 8355319

Klein-Schwartz W, Benson BE, Lee SC, et al: Comparison of citalopram and other selective serotonin reuptake inhibitor ingestions in children. Clin Toxicol (Phila) 50(5):418–423, 2012 22506805

Nazarian DJ, Broder JS, Thiessen MEW, et al: Clinical policy: critical issues in the diagnosis and management of the adult psychiatric patient in the emergency department. Ann Emerg Med 69(4):480–498, 2017 28335913

Okusa MD, Crystal LJ: Clinical manifestations and management of acute lithium intoxication. Am J Med 97(4):383–389, 1994 7942943

Suchard JR: Assessing physostigmine's contraindication in cyclic antidepressant ingestions. J Emerg Med 25(2):185–191, 2003 12902007

Chapter 13

Polypharmacy and Acute Side Effects

Sweta Bhoopatiraju, B.S.
Marissa Hirsch, M.D.
Harjinderpal Singh, B.S., B.Ed.
George Grossberg, M.D.

Polypharmacy, most frequently defined as a single patient's use of five or more concomitant medications daily, is increasingly common in the United States (Masnoon et al. 2017). This is especially true for older adults (i.e., 65 years and older), who are at an increased risk for using multiple prescriptions and over-the-counter drugs. In a national cross-sectional study from 2009 to 2016, 65.1% of older adults were prescribed at least two drugs, and 36.8% were prescribed more than five (Young et al. 2021). Although pharmacotherapy can substantially improve patients' quality of life, side effects and drug-drug and/or drug-disease interactions can result in decreased therapeutic effect or, frequently, even adverse drug events (ADEs). Common ADEs include falls, orthostatic hypotension, delirium, renal failure, and gastrointestinal and intracranial bleeds (Lavan and Gallagher 2016).

The increased burden of polypharmacy can be explained in part by age-related pharmacokinetic and pharmacodynamic changes. Older adults have a reduction in lean muscle mass and water content and an increase in proportion of total body fat, influencing the volume of distribution, and therefore risk of toxicity, of many drugs. CNS changes also occur, with relative atrophy of the substantia nigra and cortical thinning associated with decreased synaptic connections causing increased susceptibility to drug-induced parkinsonism and delirium, respectively. Senescence also causes glomerular filtration rate and total albumin level to decline, affecting drug clearance (Lavan and Gallagher 2016).

Recognition and Detection

The American Geriatrics Society Beers Criteria for Potentially Inappropriate Medication Use in Older Adults (65 years and older) are helpful in identifying medications with significant adverse side-effect profiles and drug-drug interactions for which the risks of use may outweigh the benefits in this population (2019 American Geriatrics Society Beers Criteria® Update Expert Panel 2019). The list of medications to avoid and use with caution in certain conditions (fall risk, dementia) is extensive and includes many medications used in psychiatric practice.

Culprit Medications

Anticholinergics

Among patients with polypharmacy, anticholinergic drugs are among the most common (Al Rihani et al. 2021). Depending on disease and clinical context, 11.3%–44.5% of patients have high anticholinergic load (Cross et al. 2016; Mantri et al. 2019).

Anticholinergic drugs are used in the elderly population for medical issues such as urinary dysfunction, Parkinson's disease, and irritable bowel syndrome. They enact their effects by acting on central and/or peripheral muscarinic receptors. Of the five subtypes of muscarinic receptors (M_1 to M_5), the adverse side effects of anticholinergics are hypothesized to be due to their antagonistic effects on M_1, M_2, and M_4 receptors. M_1 receptors are mostly located in the CNS and play an important role in executive functions and episodic memory. M_2 receptors are associated with memory processing, and M_4 receptors are important in regulating acetylcholine levels (López-Álvarez et al. 2019). CNS side effects of anticholinergics in older adults include confusion, sedation, impaired concentration, delirium, restlessness, agitation, ataxia, and falls (López-Álvarez et al. 2019). Peripheral nervous system effects include constipation, xerostomia, urinary retention, blurry vision, tachycardia, and mydriasis.

Many commonly prescribed drugs have anticholinergic effects, even if that is not their main therapeutic mechanism of action. Examples of commonly prescribed drugs with anticholinergic effects include antihistamines, tricyclic antidepressants, antipsychotics, antiepileptics, antiparkinsonian agents, and urological medications used to treat overactive bladder (López-Álvarez et al. 2019).

When several of these drugs are taken concomitantly, the combined anticholinergic effect, or *anticholinergic burden*, can be profound. To quantify this cumulative risk, the Anticholinergic Cognitive Burden Scale was developed (Boustani et al. 2008). This measure includes a point system for specific anticholinergic medications that correlates with an associated decrease in the Mini-Mental State Examination score and risk of premature death (Fox et al. 2011).

Benzodiazepines

Benzodiazepines are commonly prescribed anxiolytics in the older adult population. In 2008, approximately 8.7% of patients age 65 or older in the United States were prescribed a benzodiazepine, with more than a third of all benzodiazepine prescriptions being for long-term use (120 days or longer). Of patients with long-term-use prescriptions, older adults accounted for the greatest proportion (Olfson et al. 2015). With regard to polypharmacy in the elderly, only one-third of benzodiazepine prescriptions are considered appropriate, with the most common reason being excessive duration or dosage (Airagnes et al. 2016).

Benzodiazepines are positive allosteric modulators of the $GABA_A$ receptor complex, which is a ligand-gated, chloride-selective ion channel. Because GABA is an inhibitory neurotransmitter, benzodiazepines reduce neuronal excitability, which can cause a calming effect on the brain. As a result, benzodiazepines are commonly used to treat anxiety, insomnia, spasticity, and epilepsy (Griffin et al. 2013).

Benzodiazepines can cause a variety of adverse side effects. Benzodiazepine side effects at low doses include sedation, lethargy, and fatigue. At high doses, benzodiazepines can lead to falls, dizziness, vertigo, impaired motor coordination, blurry vision, and slurred speech. Over time, benzodiazepines can accumulate in the CNS and cause impaired thinking, disorientation, and confusion. This is especially concerning in the older adult population because benzodiazepines are lipophilic and have a larger volume of distribution in older compared with younger patients. As a result, benzodiazepines have a prolonged half-life and are more likely to cause sedation, confusion, disorientation, and delirium. In addition, benzodiazepines' negative effects can be attenuated or potentiated by drugs that affect the liver's cytochrome P450 system (i.e., phenytoin, rifampin, carbamazepine, some antifungals) because benzodiazepines are metabolized by the P450 system before they are glucuronidated and eliminated through the kidneys (Griffin et al. 2013).

Opioids and Narcotic Analgesics

Chronic pain is highly prevalent in older adults and can significantly impair patients' quality of life; approximately 45%–85% of older individuals have complaints about persistent pain (Guerriero 2017). To manage pain, opioids are often prescribed. Polypharmacy is quite common among adults taking opioids, with more than 20% of opioid users in a 2014 Medicare Part D analysis taking more than 10 concurrent medications (Medicare Payment Advisory Committee 2015). In the geriatric population, 75% of patients with CNS polypharmacy used opioids (Gerlach et al. 2017). Opioids exert their effects through the μ, δ, and κ receptors by closing N-type voltage-gated calcium channels and opening calcium-dependent potassium channels, resulting in hyperpolarization and neuronal inhibition in both the peripheral nervous system and the CNS (Bovill 1997).

Opioid use among older adults increases the risk for a variety of adverse events. ADEs in older adults include impaired coordination and falls, sedation, confusion and delirium, constipation, urinary retention, and respiratory and CNS depression (Chau et al. 2008).

Antipsychotics

Polypharmacy involving antipsychotic drugs is common in the United States, with a prevalence of 27.1% in 2017 (Boskailo et al. 2017). This often occurs for several reasons, including clinician dissatisfaction with primary antipsychotics, quick therapeutic response, and severe course of illness. However, a meta-analysis of 31 studies comparing the use of two or more antipsychotics with monotherapy showed that augmentation resulted in increased symptom reduction, but this was true only in open-label and low-quality trials (Galling et al. 2016).

Antipsychotic drugs can have significant side effects in geriatric patients. In patients with dementia, antipsychotic use increases the risk for death, cerebrovascular adverse events, parkinsonism, sedation, gait disturbance, cognitive decline, and pneumonia. Low-potency first-generation antipsychotics (i.e., chlorpromazine, thioridazine) and some second-generation antipsychotics (i.e., clozapine, olanzapine) have anticholinergic side-effect profiles and can cause these concerns. High-potency first-generation antipsychotics such as haloperidol and fluphenazine and high-potency second-generation antipsychotics such as risperidone have increased affinity for dopamine receptors compared with their low-potency counterparts and are more likely to cause extrapyramidal symptoms, neuroleptic malignant syndrome, dystonia, and tardive dyskinesia. In the case of clozapine, side effects (particularly agranulocytosis, sedation, neutropenia) are a major reason for discontinuation of the drug, especially when the drug is titrated quickly (Masand 2000). Some evidence suggests that antipsychotics may contribute to progressive decline and increased risk for dementia as well, although large randomized controlled trials are needed to elucidate this further (MacKenzie et al. 2018).

Assessment

When assessing for polypharmacy, it is important to obtain a list of and review all medications and over-the-counter remedies that the patient is taking. The medication regimen must then be assessed for potentially inappropriate prescribing by referencing the American Geriatrics Society Beers Criteria for Potentially Inappropriate Medication Use in Older Adults (2019 American Geriatrics Society Beers Criteria® Update Expert Panel 2019). Side effects and drug interactions resulting from substance misuse in the older adult population, which is often underdiagnosed by clinicians, also must be considered because nearly 1 million older adults had a substance use disorder in 2018 (Substance Abuse and Mental Health Services Administration 2019). A blood alcohol level and urine drug screen should be ordered if the clinician suspects substance use disorder (Moeller et al. 2008).

Management

Because older adults can have multiple medical comorbidities that affect their quality of life, it is important to find an appropriate balance between treating medical and psychiatric conditions and avoiding medication-related harm. Management of older adult patients should thus involve 1) a determination of treatment goals, 2) a review of all medications the patient is taking, 3) detection of potentially inappropriate prescriptions, 4) discontinuation of inappropriate medications, and 5) institution of appropriate nonpharmacological treatment and/or safer alternative medications (Grossberg et al. 2017).

Because older adults often have extensive medication lists, reviewing and discontinuing inappropriate medications can be daunting. Rational deprescribing is one approach (Grossberg et al. 2017) that includes the following strategies:

- Discontinuing unnecessary medications and medications that have not been beneficial or have been only marginally beneficial
- Stopping medications that were effective but not expected to provide continued benefit
- Reducing the dosage of medication if a significant change in the patient's health occurs
- Avoiding fixed combinations of medications when possible
- Reducing the frequency of medication administration
- Switching medication formulation from short-acting (multiple times daily) to long-acting (once daily) to improve adherence if no adverse side effects or cost issues exist

Follow-Up Management

After deprescribing, it is important to monitor the patient for rebound symptoms of the primary disease and withdrawal symptoms (Turner et al. 2017). Adjustments to medications and treatment regimens should be made as necessary via shared decision-making.

Conclusion

Polypharmacy, which typically describes the concurrent use of five or more drugs, can profoundly affect older patients. Older adults are at increased risk for ADEs because of the physiological changes that result from aging and the subsequent effect of drugs and drug-drug interactions. Culprit drugs can be recognized by referencing the American Geriatrics Society Beers Criteria, which list commonly prescribed medications that should be avoided or used with caution in older adults—most notably, anticholinergic drugs, benzodiazepines, opioids, and antipsychotics. To manage polypharmacy, clinicians should engage in shared decision-making with patients to determine treatment goals, review all their medications carefully, detect potentially inappropriate medications, deprescribe, and implement nonpharmacological treatment and/or safer medications. Patients should always be monitored for both symptoms of primary disease and drug withdrawal symptoms.

Key Points

Polypharmacy is most commonly defined as the prescription of five or more concurrent medications and can lead to significant adverse drug events in the older adult population.

To detect drugs that put patients at high risk for adverse drug events, the American Geriatrics Society Beers Criteria can be referenced.

Anticholinergic drugs, benzodiazepines, opioids, and antipsychotics should be avoided in older adults unless necessary.

Management of polypharmacy should include consideration of treatment goals, a thorough review of all medications, detection of potentially inappropriate medications, rational deprescribing, and the implementation of nonpharmacological treatment and/or safer medications.

References

2019 American Geriatrics Society Beers Criteria® Update Expert Panel: American Geriatrics Society 2019 updated AGS Beers Criteria® for Potentially Inappropriate Medication Use in Older Adults. J Am Geriatr Soc 67(4):674–694, 2019 30693946

Airagnes G, Pelissolo A, Lavallée M, et al: Benzodiazepine misuse in the elderly: risk factors, consequences, and management. Curr Psychiatry Rep 18(10):89, 2016 27549604

Al Rihani SB, Deodhar M, Darakjian LI, et al: Quantifying anticholinergic burden and sedative load in older adults with polypharmacy: a systematic review of risk scales and models. Drugs Aging 38(11):977–994, 2021 34751922

Boskailo E, Malkoc A, McCurry DB, et al: Assessment of inpatient psychiatric readmission risk among patients discharged on an antipsychotic polypharmacy regimen: a retrospective cohort study. Acta Med Acad 46(2):133–144, 2017 29338277

Boustani MA, Campbell NL, Munger S, et al: Impact of anticholinergics on the aging brain: a review and practical application. Aging Health 4(3):311–320, 2008

Bovill JG: Mechanisms of actions of opioids and non-steroidal anti-inflammatory drugs. Eur J Anaesthesiol Suppl 15:9–15, 1997 9202932

Chau DL, Walker V, Pai L, Cho LM: Opiates and elderly: use and side effects. Clin Interv Aging 3(2):273–278, 2008 18686750

Cross AJ, George J, Woodward MC, et al: Potentially inappropriate medications and anticholinergic burden in older people attending memory clinics in Australia. Drugs Aging 33(1):37–44, 2016 26645294

Fox C, Richardson K, Maidment ID, et al: Anticholinergic medication use and cognitive impairment in the older population: the medical research council cognitive function and ageing study. J Am Geriatr Soc 59(8):1477–1483, 2011 21707557

Galling B, Roldán A, Rietschel L, et al: Safety and tolerability of antipsychotic co-treatment in patients with schizophrenia: results from a systematic review and meta-analysis of randomized controlled trials. Expert Opin Drug Saf 15(5):591–612, 2016 26967126

Gerlach LB, Olfson M, Kales HC, Maust DT: Opioids and other central nervous system-active polypharmacy in older adults in the United States. J Am Geriatr Soc 65(9):2052–2056, 2017 28467623

Griffin CE III, Kaye AM, Bueno FR, Kaye AD: Benzodiazepine pharmacology and central nervous system-mediated effects. Ochsner J 13(2):214–223, 2013 23789008

Grossberg GT, Desai AK, Waun J: Psychiatric aspects of rational deprescribing, in Psychiatric Consultation in Long-Term Care: A Guide for Healthcare Professionals, 2nd Edition. Cambridge, UK, Cambridge University Press, 2017, pp 330–360

Guerriero F: Guidance on opioids prescribing for the management of persistent non-cancer pain in older adults. World J Clin Cases 5(3):73–81, 2017 28352631

Lavan AH, Gallagher P: Predicting risk of adverse drug reactions in older adults. Ther Adv Drug Saf 7(1):11–22, 2016 26834959

López-Álvarez J, Sevilla-Llewellyn-Jones J, Agüera-Ortiz L: Anticholinergic drugs in geriatric psychopharmacology. Front Neurosci 13:1309, 2019 31866817

MacKenzie NE, Kowalchuk C, Agarwal SM, et al: Antipsychotics, metabolic adverse effects, and cognitive function in schizophrenia. Front Psychiatry 9:622, 2018 30568606

Mantri S, Fullard M, Gray SL, et al: Patterns of dementia treatment and frank prescribing errors in older adults with Parkinson disease. JAMA Neurol 76(1):41–49, 2019 30285047

Masand PS: Side effects of antipsychotics in the elderly. J Clin Psychiatry 61(Suppl 8):43–49, discussion 50–51, 2000 10811243

Masnoon N, Shakib S, Kalisch-Ellett L, et al: What is polypharmacy? A systematic review of definitions. BMC Geriatr 17(1):230, 2017 29017448

Medicare Payment Advisory Committee: Polypharmacy and opioid use among Medicare Part D enrollees, in Report to Congress: Medicare and the Health Care Delivery System. June 2015. Available at: www.medpac.gov/wp-content/uploads/import_data/scrape_files/docs/default-source/reports/chapter-5-polypharmacy-and-opioid-use-among-medicare-part-d-enrollees-june-2015-report-.pdf. Accessed October 7, 2021.

Moeller KE, Lee KC, Kissack JC: Urine drug screening: practical guide for clinicians [erratum in: Mayo Clin Proc 83(7):851, 2008]. Mayo Clin Proc 83(1):66–76, 2008 18174009

Olfson M, King M, Schoenbaum M: Benzodiazepine use in the United States. JAMA Psychiatry 72(2):136–142, 2015 25517224

Substance Abuse and Mental Health Services Administration: Results from the 2018 National Survey on Drug Use and Health: detailed tables. Center for Behavioral Health Statistics and Quality, Substance Abuse and Mental Health Services Administration, 2019. Available at: www.samhsa.gov/data/report/2018-nsduh-detailed-tables. Accessed July 7, 2022.

Turner JP, Shakib S, Bell JS: Is my older cancer patient on too many medications? J Geriatr Oncol 8(2):77–81, 2017 27840102

Young EH, Pan S, Yap AG, et al: Polypharmacy prevalence in older adults seen in United States physician offices from 2009 to 2016. PLoS One 16(8):e0255642, 2021 34343225

Chapter 14

Pregnancy and Use of Psychotropic Medication

Katherine Taljan, M.D.
Adele C. Viguera, M.D., M.P.H.

Prenatal psychiatric illness is common and associated with adverse maternal and neonatal outcomes. Decisions about psychotropic medication use during pregnancy should take into account risks of in utero medication exposure as well as risks of untreated maternal illness.

Depression and anxiety affect 15%–20% of pregnant women. Untreated mood and anxiety disorders during pregnancy are associated with many adverse maternal and neonatal outcomes, including poor adherence to medical care, worsening of maternal medical conditions, tobacco and substance use, preterm birth, and low birth weight. Women with mood and anxiety disorders during pregnancy are also more likely to develop postpartum depression, which may impair maternal-infant bonding and child development or result in maternal suicide or infanticide (Betcher and Wisner 2020).

Psychotropic medications are commonly discontinued during pregnancy, often because of concerns about teratogenic or developmental effects of in utero medication exposure (Raffi et al. 2019). Although there are reassuring data on the reproductive safety of some commonly prescribed psychotropic medications, robust studies of the effects of in utero exposure to many psychotropic medications have not been conducted (Betcher and Wisner 2020). Under the updated Pregnancy and Lactation Labeling Rule implemented by the FDA in 2015, the system of classifying medications into lettered categories (A, B, C, D, X) was replaced with a narrative summary of risks and relevant data (Raffi et al. 2019).

Recognition and Detection

Identification of medication exposures during pregnancy may be obtained through the patient interview and review of medical records.

Culprit Medications

Selective Serotonin Reuptake Inhibitors

A large body of data suggests that selective serotonin reuptake inhibitors (SSRIs), which include fluoxetine, paroxetine, sertraline, escitalopram, citalopram, and fluvoxamine, are relatively safe for use during pregnancy. SSRI use is associated with small risks of preterm birth (<37 weeks' gestation), low birth weight, and postpartum hemorrhage (Betcher and Wisner 2020; Raffi et al. 2019). A clear link between SSRI use and miscarriage has not been established because of the difficulty of controlling for confounding factors such as maternal age and tobacco use (Raffi et al. 2019). Most SSRIs are not associated with major congenital malformations in well-controlled studies (Betcher and Wisner 2020), with the exception of paroxetine, which has been associated with risk of fetal cardiac defects in some, but not all, studies (Huybrechts et al. 2014). Fewer data are available for fluvoxamine relative to other SSRIs, but available data do not show an increased risk of congenital malformations (Raffi et al. 2019).

In the first days to weeks after delivery, up to 30% of infants exposed to SSRIs in utero show transient symptoms of neonatal adaptation, including tachypnea, hypoglycemia, temperature instability, irritability, weak cry, and tremulousness. The severity of these symptoms varies widely, although some infants may require admission to the neonatal intensive care unit (Betcher and Wisner 2020). SSRI use is also associated with an increased risk for persistent pulmonary hypertension of the newborn (PPHN), which may cause severe respiratory failure or neonatal death. However, the absolute risk of PPHN following SSRI exposure is small, with recent meta-analyses finding an absolute risk difference of 0.619 per 1,000 live births and a number needed to harm of 1,615 women (Ng et al. 2019). Limited data suggest that SSRI exposure is not associated with changes in behavioral or cognitive development (Raffi et al. 2019).

Serotonin-Norepinephrine Reuptake Inhibitors

Serotonin-norepinephrine reuptake inhibitors include venla-faxine and its metabolite desvenlafaxine, as well as duloxe-tine and levomilnacipran. Currently, data on the safety of desvenlafaxine or levomilnacipran use during pregnancy are insufficient. Available data on prenatal exposure to venlafax-ine and duloxetine do not show a consistent association with miscarriage or structural malformations. Rates of preterm birth, poor neonatal adaptation, and PPHN may be similar to those of SSRIs. Limited data suggest that venlafaxine exposure is not associated with changes in behavioral or cognitive devel-opment through early childhood. Serotonin-norepinephrine reuptake inhibitor use during pregnancy is associated with a significantly increased risk of gestational hypertension, par-ticularly at higher medication doses (Raffi et al. 2019).

Bupropion, Mirtazapine, and Trazodone

Limited data suggest that bupropion is relatively safe for use in pregnancy, with risks of spontaneous abortion similar to those of other antidepressants and no significant increases in rates of congenital malformations, preterm delivery, or low birth weight. Limited reports suggest that mirtazapine and trazo-done are not associated with an increased risk of miscarriage or major congenital malformations, but further research is needed to better characterize the safety profile of these medications. Further research is also needed to assess the risk of neonatal ad-aptation and other outcomes associated with antenatal use of bupropion, mirtazapine, and trazodone (Raffi et al. 2019).

Tricyclic Antidepressants

Tricyclic antidepressants (TCAs) include amitriptyline, nor-triptyline, imipramine, desipramine, amoxapine, and dox-epin. Most studies indicate that TCAs are similar to SSRIs with respect to risk for spontaneous abortion and structural malformations, as well as for neonatal adaptation syndrome and child development outcomes. The α-adrenergic effects of some TCAs may exacerbate antenatal orthostatic hypoten-sion (Raffi et al. 2019).

Lithium

Exposure to lithium in the first trimester has been associated with an increased risk of congenital cardiac malformations, including right ventricular outflow tract anomalies, although some data suggest that this risk may be more modest than previously believed (Poels et al. 2018). An analysis of more than 1.3 million pregnancies found that lithium exposure in the first trimester was associated with an increased risk of cardiac malformations on the order of 1 additional case per 100 pregnancies. This same study found that the risk of cardiac malformations was related to lithium dosage, with the least risk seen for dosages at or below 600 mg daily (RR=1.11; 95% CI=0.46–2.64) and the greatest risk seen for dosages greater than 900 mg daily (RR=3.22; 95% CI=1.47–7.02) (Patorno et al. 2017).

Lamotrigine

Studies of lamotrigine-exposed pregnancies have reported that rates of miscarriage, stillbirth, preterm deliveries, and small for gestational age newborns are similar to those observed in the general population. Studies have also found no increased risk of congenital malformations between pregnant women exposed to lamotrigine and disease-matched control subjects (Tomson et al. 2018). Because of estrogen-induced metabolism, lamotrigine doses may need to be increased during pregnancy to maintain mood stability (Betcher and Wisner 2020).

Valproic Acid

Prenatal exposure to valproic acid is highly associated with major malformations, including neural tube defects, midface hypoplasia, congenital heart defects, cleft lip and palate, and microcephaly, along with increased risk for in utero growth restriction and neurodevelopmental outcomes such as intellectual disability and autism spectrum disorder (Tomson et al. 2018). According to expert consensus, valproic acid should be discontinued during pregnancy (Anmella et al. 2019).

Carbamazepine, Oxcarbazepine, and Topiramate

Prenatal carbamazepine exposure is associated with an increased risk for major congenital malformations, including neural tube defects, and should be avoided in pregnancy. Reproductive safety data are limited for oxcarbazepine and topiramate (Betcher and Wisner 2020; Tomson et al. 2018).

Antipsychotics

Available studies suggest that antipsychotics are relatively safe for use in pregnancy, although more research is still needed (Betcher and Wisner 2020). A large study of 1.3 million pregnancies found that when researchers controlled for confounding factors, exposure to typical or atypical antipsychotics in the first trimester of pregnancy was not associated with a significantly increased risk for major congenital malformations. A small increased risk in overall congenital malformations and cardiac malformations was found for risperidone independent of all measured confounders (Huybrechts et al. 2016).

Psychostimulants

Research on the safety of psychostimulants is mixed. A study of 1.8 million pregnancies in the United States and 2.6 million pregnancies in Nordic countries found that first-trimester exposure to amphetamines was not associated with a significantly increased risk for overall congenital malformations or cardiac malformations. The same study found a small but significant increased risk of cardiac malformations associated with first-trimester exposure to methylphenidate (Huybrechts et al. 2018). Psychostimulant use also has been associated with modest increases in risk of preeclampsia, preterm birth, and placental abruption (Cohen et al. 2017).

Atomoxetine

Limited data suggest that atomoxetine exposure is not associated with preeclampsia, preterm birth, or placental abruption, but other safety data are sparse (Cohen et al. 2017).

Benzodiazepines

Recent research suggests that risks of benzodiazepine exposure in pregnancy may be more modest than previously thought, although still present (Betcher and Wisner 2020). A recent study of more than 400,000 pregnancies found that benzodiazepine use in early pregnancy was associated with an increased risk for spontaneous abortion, even after controlling for confounding factors, including maternal mental illness (Sheehy et al. 2019). A meta-analysis of available literature found no significant association between prenatal benzodiazepine use and overall congenital malformations or cardiac malformations. However, the same study found that concurrent use of benzodiazepines and antidepressants significantly increased the risk for congenital malformations (Grigoriadis et al. 2019). Prenatal exposure to benzodiazepines has also been associated with neonatal adaptation symptoms, including respiratory distress, infections, cardiac abnormalities, and neurobehavioral changes (Betcher and Wisner 2020).

Assessment

Assessment of the pregnant patient should begin with a comprehensive psychiatric evaluation, including a review of the psychiatric history and the presence of suicidal ideation, high-risk behavior, or functional impairment. Rating scales, such as the Edinburgh Postnatal Depression Scale, can be used to screen for symptoms of perinatal depression but do not take the place of expert clinical evaluation. The presence of medical comorbidities, including those related to pregnancy, should be assessed. A detailed medication history should include past medication trials as well as compliance with and response to current medications.

The clinician should evaluate the patient's risk for relapse during pregnancy. Women with preexisting major depression are at high risk for illness recurrence during pregnancy, particularly if they have experienced more than four lifetime episodes or have a history of depression lasting more than 5 years. Women with major depressive disorder who discontinue psychotropic medication during pregnancy experience higher relapse rates than do women who continue medications (Cohen et al. 2006). Among women with bipolar disorder, approximately 70% experience at least one recurrence during pregnancy. Women who discontinue mood stabilizers are twice as likely to relapse while also having a fourfold shorter time to first recurrence and fivefold longer duration of illness (Viguera et al. 2007).

Management

Decisions about medication changes should balance the risks of psychotropic medication exposure against the risks of exposure to untreated maternal mental illness.

Patient Education and Counseling

Clinicians should present pregnant patients with the most up-to-date information on the risks of in utero medication exposure, along with the risks of untreated maternal mental illness. Patients should be counseled that abrupt discontinuation of psychotropic medications may lead to adverse physical and psychological effects, including the development of suicidal ideation (Cohen et al. 2006; Viguera et al. 2007).

Mild Illness

For patients with a history of mild illness, medication discontinuation during pregnancy may be appropriate, particularly if it is the patient's preference. Patients with a history of mild anxiety or depression who discontinue medication may benefit from psychotherapy or peer support groups both during and after pregnancy. Because abrupt medication discontinuation increases the risk for relapse, it may be beneficial to taper medications over several weeks, with careful monitoring for symptom recurrence. Ongoing monitoring of mental health symptoms should continue throughout pregnancy and the postpartum period. Patients should be counseled on the risks of symptom relapse and the option to resume medication during pregnancy.

Moderate to Severe Illness

For cases of moderate to severe illness, the risks of relapse or functional impairment from illness may be more substantial than the risks of continuing medication. In some cases, changing from a medication with less available safety data to one that has been more extensively studied may be appropriate. Highly teratogenic medications such as valproic acid and carbamazepine should be replaced by medications with a more favorable safety profile, such as lamotrigine or an antipsychotic. However, there is no expert consensus on whether valproic acid or carbamazepine should be discontinued abruptly or tapered, so clinical judgment should be used in individual cases (Anmella et al. 2019). Reduction of polypharmacy and use of the lowest effective doses should be attempted in order to further reduce medication exposures (Betcher and Wisner 2020).

Difficult Cases

For patients who have not responded to trials of well-studied medications, it may be justified to continue a medication with relatively fewer safety data. For patients maintained on lithium, a dose reduction to 600 mg or less in the first trimester may reduce the risk of congenital malformations. Lithium doses may need to be increased in the second and third trimesters because of increases in blood volume and glomerular filtration rate (Poels et al. 2018). Twice- or thrice-daily dosing can be used in later pregnancy to stabilize plasma concentrations (Betcher and Wisner 2020).

Folic acid supplementation reduces the risk of neural tube defects, and some experts recommend dosages between 500 µg and 5 mg daily for women taking antiepileptic drugs. However, use of folic acid as prophylaxis in pregnant women undergoing anticonvulsant treatment has not been systemically studied (Stephen et al. 2019). Patients taking lithium or exposed to valproic acid during pregnancy should be offered level II fetal ultrasonography with detailed cardiac evaluation around 20 weeks' gestation (Poels et al. 2018), which may provide reassurance about fetal development or aid in planning for neonatal care after birth.

Follow-Up Management

Selective Serotonin Reuptake Inhibitors

Infants exposed to SSRIs in utero should be observed directly following delivery for signs of poor neonatal adaptation. SSRIs generally can be continued during lactation, and exposure to SSRIs through lactation is typically less than with transplacental exposure (Betcher and Wisner 2020).

Lamotrigine

Because of changes in estrogen levels following parturition, lamotrigine should be reduced to prepregnancy doses within 10 days postpartum. Experts recommend that if the lamotrigine dose was increased four or more times during pregnancy, then the dose should be decreased by 20%–25% immediately on delivery to avoid toxicity (Betcher and Wisner 2020).

Lithium

If lithium was continued during pregnancy, maternal lithium levels should be measured 24 hours after delivery (Poels et al. 2018). Because of fluid shifts and metabolic changes, lithium levels may need to be adjusted immediately after delivery to avoid lithium toxicity, particularly if doses were increased later in pregnancy (Betcher and Wisner 2020).

Newborns who were exposed to lithium in utero should be directly observed postdelivery, and umbilical cord blood samples should also be tested for lithium blood level, thyroid-stimulating hormone, and free thyroxine. Because infants exposed to higher lithium concentrations (>0.64 mEq/L) at the time of delivery are at risk for lower Apgar scores, longer hospital stays, and higher rates of CNS and neuromuscular complications, some experts recommend discontinuing lithium 24–48 hours prior to delivery (Betcher and Wisner 2020). However, because this strategy may increase the risk for maternal relapse without significantly changing neonatal outcomes, other experts recommend continuing lithium along with measuring levels and ensuring adequate peripartum fluid management (Poels et al. 2018).

If lithium was discontinued during pregnancy, experts recommend resumption immediately after delivery to protect against relapse of bipolar disorder. In the first month postpartum, a higher therapeutic level (0.8–1.0 mmol/L) may optimize relapse prevention. Because of the lack of sufficient information on infant lithium levels and consequences of exposure through breast milk, breastfeeding while taking lithium is discouraged by many experts and various national guidelines (Poels et al. 2018). However, because lithium excretion into breast milk is variable and reports exist of infants who were breastfed during maternal lithium therapy without signs of toxicity or developmental problems, some mothers may choose to breastfeed while maintained on lithium. In these cases, close pediatric follow-up and periodic monitoring of infant lithium serum level, thyroid, and renal function tests are recommended (National Library of Medicine 2021).

Other Medications

Clinicians can use resources such as the National Institutes of Health Drugs and Lactation Database (www.ncbi.nlm.nih.gov/books/NBK501922) to access up-to-date information on the safety of other psychotropic medications in lactation.

Conclusion

Although psychiatric illness is common during pregnancy and carries risks for poor maternal and neonatal outcomes, appropriate medication management can prevent symptom recurrence, maintain maternal well-being, and reduce the risks to fetal health and development.

Key Points

Women with preexisting mental illness are at high risk for relapse during pregnancy.

Untreated maternal mental illness is a risk factor for poor maternal and neonatal outcomes, including preterm birth, low birth weight, and postpartum depression.

Abrupt discontinuation of psychotropic medications may lead to adverse physical and psychiatric symptoms, including the emergence of suicidal ideation.

Reproductive safety data are available for some, but not all, psychotropic medications.

Decisions about psychotropic medication use during pregnancy should take into account the risks of in utero medication exposure and the risks of untreated maternal illness.

General management strategies include reduction of polypharmacy and use of the lowest effective doses of medications with good safety profiles.

Highly teratogenic medications such as valproic acid and carbamazepine should be discontinued during pregnancy and replaced, if needed, with other medications.

Use of low-dose lithium during pregnancy may be justified in cases of severe bipolar disorder with poor response to other medications.

Infants exposed to psychotropic medications in utero should be observed directly after birth for signs of poor neonatal adaptation, with further testing as indicated.

References

Anmella G, Pacchiarotti, I, Cubała WJ, et al: Expert advice on the management of valproate in women with bipolar disorder at childbearing age. Eur Neuropsychopharmacol 29(11):1199–1212, 2019 31590972

Betcher HK, Wisner KL: Psychotropic treatment during pregnancy: research synthesis and clinical care principles. J Womens Health 29(3):310–318, 2020 31800350

Cohen JM, Hernández-Díaz S, Bateman BT, et al: Placental complications associated with psychostimulant use in pregnancy. Obstet Gynecol 130(6):1192–1201, 2017 29112657

Cohen LS, Altshuler LL, Harlow BL, et al: Relapse of major depression during pregnancy in women who maintain or discontinue antidepressant treatment. JAMA 295(5):499–507, 2006 16449615

Grigoriadis S, Graves L, Peer M, et al: Benzodiazepine use during pregnancy alone or in combination with an antidepressant and congenital malformations: systematic review and meta-analysis. J Clin Psychiatry 80(4):18r12412, 2019 31294935

Huybrechts KF, Palmsten K, Avorn J, et al: Antidepressant use in pregnancy and the risk of cardiac defects. N Engl J Med 370(25):2397–2407, 2014 24941178

Huybrechts KF, Hernández-Díaz S, Patorno E, et al: Antipsychotic use in pregnancy and the risk for congenital malformations. JAMA Psychiatry 73(9):938–946, 2016 27540849

Huybrechts KF, Bröms G, Christensen LB, et al: Association between methylphenidate and amphetamine use in pregnancy and risk of congenital malformations: a cohort study from the International Pregnancy Safety Study Consortium. JAMA Psychiatry 75(2):167–175, 2018 29238795

National Library of Medicine: Lithium, in Drugs and Lactation Database (LactMed). 2021. Available at: www.ncbi.nlm.nih.gov/books/NBK501922. Accessed November 9, 2022.

Ng QX, Venkatanarayanan N, Ho C, et al: Selective serotonin reuptake inhibitors and persistent pulmonary hypertension of the newborn: an update meta-analysis. J Womens Health 28(3):331–338, 2019 30407100

Patorno E, Huybrechts KF, Bateman BT, et al: Lithium use in pregnancy and the risk of cardiac malformations. N Engl J Med 376(23):2245–2254, 2017 28591541

Poels EMP, Bijma HH, Galbally M, Bergink V: Lithium during pregnancy and after delivery: a review. Int J Bipolar Disord 6(1):26, 2018 30506447

Raffi ER, Nonacs R, Cohen LS: Safety of psychotropic medications during pregnancy. Clin Perinatol 46(2):215–234, 2019 31010557

Sheehy O, Zhao JP, Bérard A: Association between incident exposure to benzodiazepines in early pregnancy and risk of spontaneous abortion. JAMA Psychiatry 76(9):948–957, 2019 31090881

Stephen LJ, Harden C, Tomson T, Brodie MJ: Management of epilepsy in women. Lancet Neurol 18(5):481–491, 2019 30857949

Tomson T, Battino D, Bonizzoni E, et al: Comparative risk of major congenital malformations with eight different antiepileptic drugs: a prospective cohort study of the EURAP registry. Lancet Neurol 17(6):530–538, 2018 29680205

Viguera AC, Whitfield T, Baldessarini RJ, et al: Risk of recurrence in women with bipolar disorder during pregnancy: prospective study of mood stabilizer discontinuation. Am J Psychiatry 164(12):1817–1824, quiz 1923, 2007 18056236

Chapter 15

Seizure Risk Management

Nicholas A. Mischel, M.D., Ph.D.

Having a seizure usually implies a generalized tonic-clonic seizure (GTCS) event such as an *epileptic* or *grand mal* seizure. These are very impressive, dramatic, and frightening experiences. One GTCS event causes lasting damage only very rarely. For clinicians, the focus is on recognition and assessment to prevent further events from occurring in unsafe contexts such as driving or operating heavy machinery.

In the normal physiological state, charged ions (Na^+, K^+, Ca^{++}, Mg^{++}, Cl^-) and ion channels determine the membrane threshold of a neuron and the propensity to produce an action potential. There is a refractory period during which an action potential will not propagate. Psychoactive agents that affect electrochemical communication between neurons may carry a seizure risk through some effect on the threshold or refractory inhibition of action potentials.

Fast-acting excitatory and inhibitory inputs to neurons are mediated by glutamate and GABA, respectively. Some agents with a seizure risk act via glutamate and GABA receptors and work generally to decrease the seizure threshold. Slower-acting regulators of neuron activity and seizure threshold include cholinergic, serotonergic, adrenergic, dopaminergic, and histaminergic systems. Nearly all these classes of agents have been shown to be generally safe and effective when used in patients with seizure disorders, and the seizure risk lies in overdose or polypharmacy.

A seizure begins with a focal locus of hyperexcitation and loss of surround inhibition, both driven by increased cytosolic Ca^{++} levels. Repeated bursting can overwhelm inhibition of surrounding targets (Bromfield et al. 2006). This type of hyperactivation may be considered *epileptiform* seizure activity. In a GTCS, activation propagates locally before generalizing to bilateral areas. Robust negative feedback mechanisms prevent runaway, excitatory, and feed-forward loops from propagating across brain regions and producing seizure activity (Bromfield et al. 2006; Devinsky et al. 2018).

Recognition and Detection

Generalized Tonic-Clonic Seizure

A GTCS is a clear event with well-known features. There is sudden loss of consciousness, then tonic, uncoordinated motor movements that reflect the initial phase of seizure generalization. This phase is usually not longer than 20 seconds. The tonic phase is followed by a clonic, or convulsive, phase of rhythmic jerking movements, beginning as high-frequency, low-amplitude myoclonic jerks and progressing to high-amplitude, low-frequency myoclonic jerks. After about 1 minute of convulsions, movements decrease, and people enter a postictal phase of gradual return to full consciousness. Amnesia and autonomic phenomena (tachycardia, hypertension, flushing, diaphoresis, enuresis, encopresis, hypopnea or hyperpnea, lacrimation) are common. Eyes usually stay open. GTCS begins with a prodrome sometimes but not always.

Simple and Complex Partial Seizure

Seizure activity that does not progress to full GTCS can be divided into epileptiform and nonepileptiform types. Non-GTCS epileptiform seizures may reflect focal epileptiform seizure activity that did not spread or fully generalize as in a GTCS. A complex partial seizure causes impaired consciousness. Awareness is retained during a simple partial seizure. All partial seizures show focal neurological phenomena with unilateral motor manifestations when present.

Other Generalized Seizure Types

Some generalized seizures do not begin focally and lack convulsive motor movements such as in absence seizures in childhood. In addition, generalized tonic seizures, or *drop attacks*, can occur with structural brain pathology, including developmental disorders in Lennox-Gastaut syndrome.

Nonepileptiform Seizures

Nonepileptiform seizure events are called psychogenic, dissociative, or blackout episodes that resemble seizure activity with heterogeneous motor and sensory symptoms. Non-epileptiform seizures show no changes on an electroencephalogram (EEG) and will less commonly show localizing signs prior to generalized motor activity, and consciousness frequently stays intact. Episodes recur and last more than 2 minutes, usually up to 5 minutes. Acute stress and autonomic activation (i.e., tachycardia, hyperventilation, diaphoresis) are frequently associated with psychogenic seizure episodes. Other nonepileptiform conditions that mimic seizures include syncope, migraine headache, dyskinesia, dystonia, myoclonus, stereotypies and tics, parasomnias, and hypoglycemia.

Culprit Medications

Psychoactive agents that carry a risk of inducing GTCS generally do so via excessive activation of a mechanism that increases neuronal resting membrane potential or decreases the threshold to generate action potentials (Devinsky et al. 2018). The mechanism that affects seizure threshold may or may not be the *on-target* mechanism for therapeutic effect.

Antidepressants

Bupropion

Excessive effects of bupropion on dopamine and norepinephrine reuptake may lower the seizure threshold. The risk of seizures with monotherapy is 0.4% incidence at 300–450 mg/day in clinical trials.

Tricyclic Antidepressants

Maprotiline, imipramine, and clomipramine carry the highest risk among tricyclic antidepressants (TCAs) and antidepressants in general (Johannessen Landmark et al. 2016). TCAs can cause seizures via excessive 5-hydroxytryptamine (serotonin, 5-HT) and norepinephrine effects that lower the seizure threshold.

Serotonin-Norepinephrine Reuptake Inhibitors and Monoamine Oxidase Inhibitors

More selective antidepressants can cause seizures in overdose or combination by excessive serotonin, dopamine, and norepinephrine effects that lower the seizure threshold. With these agents there is no known risk of seizure with monotherapy; in fact, therapeutic use lowers risk (Alper et al. 2007).

Vilazodone

Some agents act by also modifying the activity of serotonin receptors rather than only increasing neurotransmitter levels (e.g., serotonin). For serotonin receptor–modifying agents such as vilazodone, seizures have occurred in case reports of single-agent overdose. The combination of actions to inhibit serotonin reuptake and partially activate the 5-HT$_{1A}$ receptor may lead to more rapid rises in synaptic serotonin than with other selective serotonin reuptake inhibitors (Baumgartner et al. 2020).

Ketamine

As an antidepressant strategy, ketamine is delivered at subanesthetic doses. Anecdotally, ketamine for procedural anesthesia may cause seizures, possibly by an acute increase in monoamine neurotransmitters, but this is unlikely to happen in healthy persons or at subanesthetic doses (Meaden and Barnes 2019).

Mood Stabilizers

Lithium can cause seizures by excessive serotonergic effects that lower the seizure threshold. Like selective serotonin reuptake inhibitors, lithium has no known risk of seizures with monotherapy. Serotonergic effects of lithium are linearly dose dependent and should be tracked with blood levels.

Antipsychotics

Seizures with typical and atypical antipsychotics are caused by excessive serotonin receptor effects that lower the seizure threshold. The risk of seizures with monotherapy is increased for some agents. For example, risk is increased with chlorpromazine and thioridazine but is decreased with haloperidol (Alper et al. 2007). Among atypical antipsychotics, clozapine, ziprasidone, olanzapine, and quetiapine have increased risk. The risk of seizures is decreased with risperidone.

Clozapine is an essential medicine for many patients and acts via diverse effects on inhibiting serotonin, dopamine, and GABA receptor subtypes. Clozapine may cause seizures by interacting with GABA_B receptors. The cumulative risk of seizures with monotherapy over 4 treatment years is 10%, and the annual risk is 4.4% with dosages greater than 600 mg/day, 2.7% with dosages from 300 to 600 mg/day, and 1% with dosages less than 300 mg/day. In order to mitigate the risk of titration-related seizure, clozapine should be titrated slowly by 25 mg/day or less (Devinsky et al. 1991).

Stimulants

Recreational and prescribed amphetamines activate trace amine–associated receptor 1 (TAAR1) to increase the release of dopamine, norepinephrine, and serotonin into the synaptic cleft. With recreational use or overdose, these drugs can cause seizures through excessive serotonin, dopamine, and norepinephrine effects that lower the seizure threshold. Seizure risk is not increased with monotherapy with amphetamines because they decrease target neuron firing rate at therapeutic doses (Ma et al. 2013). Methylphenidate showed an increased seizure risk that occurred in the first 30 days of treatment in a large Hong Kong–based population study (Man et al. 2020). Excessive effects on dopamine and norepinephrine reuptake may lower the seizure threshold, and methylphenidate increases target neuron firing rate.

Anxiolytics

Benzodiazepines

Benzodiazepines are one of the most prescribed medications in psychiatry and neurology. In general, long-acting benzodiazepines such as clonazepam and diazepam increase the seizure threshold acutely and have a low risk of seizure in withdrawal because of their very long half-lives. Very-short-acting benzodiazepines such as alprazolam, lorazepam, and oxazepam may have a risk of seizure in withdrawal, especially if there is cowithdrawal from alcohol (Ait-Daoud et al. 2018).

Buspirone

Buspirone is a serotonin receptor modifier that acts acutely to alleviate anxiety. In overdose, it can cause seizure activity in rare cases (Catalano et al. 1998).

Repetitive Transcranial Magnetic Stimulation and Psychoactive Medications

Combining repetitive transcranial magnetic stimulation (rTMS) with any of the following substances can lead to excessive cortical excitability, increasing the risk of rTMS-related seizures: stimulants, caffeine, TCAs, monoamine oxidase inhibitors, bupropion, clozapine, and steroids. rTMS delivered above 120% of the resting motor threshold may increase seizure risk. High-frequency rTMS stimulation may cause a seizure if the ratio of active stimulation to rest interval within a repeated pattern protocol is increased outside known safety limits, about 1:2. In addition, appropriate rTMS stimulation may induce seizure in the context of alcohol or benzodiazepine withdrawal and sleep deprivation (Lefaucheur et al. 2020).

Assessment

As part of the history and physical examination, vital signs, mental status, and a neurological examination should be documented. Blood levels of offending agents as well as electrolytes, urea nitrogen, and glucose should be obtained. If possible, nasal oxygen and electrocardiogram recording should be started. If convulsions do not cease after approximately 2 minutes, if vitals do not stabilize after convulsions, or if the patient does not return to consciousness after convulsions, the emergency medical response protocol for the care setting should be activated, or emergency services should be called.

Management

If seizure is induced in the context of a known precipitant, immediate management will follow rapid medical response guidelines. First, clinicians must ensure that the patient is physically safe; for example, by assisting the patient in prevention of unintentional self-harm during a seizure by helping them to the bed or floor if necessary and placing padding where appropriate during convulsions. Then, the specific acute response protocol for the current care setting should be activated. This may be a protocol specific to seizure events, a *rapid response* team, or getting help to call emergency services.

If a provoked seizure that was prolonged or atypical in nature occurred in the outpatient setting, transfer to an emergency department should be considered. Prolonged seizures (as in the case of nonconvulsive status epilepticus) are best managed in a neurospecific intensive care setting with access to an epilepsy specialist. *Status epilepticus* occurs when consciousness does not begin to return and seizure activity does not cease after 20 minutes or the patient experiences more than one GTCS within 5 minutes. Status epilepticus is a medical emergency requiring intubation.

Depending on the care setting, a provider may have the option of administering an abortive medication if epileptic seizure activity is prolonged. This may include benzodiazepines or other antiepileptic drugs, delivered intravenously or intramuscularly. Guidelines suggest intravenous lorazepam infusion followed by fosphenytoin as first-line therapy. Second-line therapies include midazolam, phenobarbital, pentobarbital, and propofol (Prasad et al. 2014).

Follow-Up Management

To confirm the etiology of the seizure, an EEG should be obtained. A 24-hour, video-recorded EEG with provocation is the gold-standard procedure to characterize event-related phenomena. A brief, or *spot*, EEG may have only limited utility, particularly in the postictal period (Smith 2005). For medication-induced epileptic seizures such as GTCS, a consultation with an epilepsy specialist regarding the risks and benefits of combining the psychoactive culprit with additional antiepileptic therapies should be considered. If an offending agent cannot be identified, a structural neuroimaging with contrast brain MRI may be indicated. In the case of nonepileptic seizures, a discussion with the patient should occur regarding the risks and benefits of prescribed and nonprescribed agents that increase the frequency of events. Medication management combined with psychotherapy is more effective for nonepileptic seizures than either strategy alone (LaFrance et al. 2014). Psychoeducation on the pathophysiology of epileptic versus nonepileptic seizures is likely to increase treatment adherence.

With respect to chronic medication management in cases of provoked seizure, essential treatments can often be continued with dose adjustment, adjunctive antiepileptic therapies, and close monitoring. Rates of psychiatric disorders are increased in patients with seizure disorders (Hesdorffer et al. 2012), and appropriate treatment usually leads to decreased seizure events. If the seizure occurred in overdose, the clinician should assess the specifics of the event and address the risks of intentional self-harm with continuing the agent. If the seizure occurred in withdrawal, the clinician should address substance use, treatment adherence, and any psychosocial barriers.

Key Points

Agents that carry a seizure risk generally affect electrochemical homeostasis at cellular and circuit levels via imbalance of excitatory and inhibitory input to a given cell or region.

Prolonged seizures (as in the case of nonconvulsive status epilepticus) are best managed in a neurospecific intensive care setting with access to an epilepsy specialist.

The risk of seizures is increased in patients with psychiatric disorders and vice versa.

Essential medicine should not be avoided merely because of increased risk of seizures.

Seizure psychoeducation is essential in follow-up management.

References

Ait-Daoud N, Hamby AS, Sharma S, et al: A review of alprazolam use, misuse, and withdrawal. J Addict Med 12(1):4–10, 2018 28777203

Alper K, Schwartz KA, Kolts RL, et al: Seizure incidence in psychopharmacological clinical trials: an analysis of Food and Drug Administration (FDA) summary basis of approval reports. Biol Psychiatry 62(4):345–354, 2007 17223086

Baumgartner K, Doering M, Schwarz E: Vilazodone poisoning: a systematic review. Clin Toxicol (Phila) 58(5):360–367, 2020 31777303

Bromfield EB, Cavazos JE, Sirven JI (eds): Basic mechanisms underlying seizures and epilepsy, in An Introduction to Epilepsy. American Epilepsy Society, 2006. Available at: www.ncbi.nlm.nih.gov/books/NBK2510. Accessed July 9, 2022.

Catalano G, Catalano MC, Hanley PF: Seizures associated with buspirone overdose: case report and literature review. Clin Neuropharmacol 21(6):347–350, 1998 9844791

Devinsky O, Honigfeld G, Patin J: Clozapine-related seizures. Neurology 41(3):369–371, 1991 2006003

Devinsky O, Vezzani A, O'Brien T, et al: Epilepsy. Nat Rev Dis Primers 4:18024, 2018

Hesdorffer DC, Ishihara L, Mynepalli L, et al: Epilepsy, suicidality, and psychiatric disorders: a bidirectional association. Ann Neurol 72(2):184–191, 2012 22887468

Johannessen Landmark C, Henning O, Johannessen SI: Proconvulsant effects of antidepressants—what is the current evidence? Epilepsy Behav 61:287–291, 2016 26926001

LaFrance WC Jr, Baird GL, Barry JJ, et al: Multicenter pilot treatment trial for psychogenic nonepileptic seizures: a randomized clinical trial. JAMA Psychiatry 71(9):997–1005, 2014 24989152

Lefaucheur JP, Aleman A, Baeken C, et al: Evidence-based guidelines on the therapeutic use of repetitive transcranial magnetic stimulation (rTMS): an update (2014–2018). Clin Neurophysiol 131(2):474–528, 2020 31901449

Ma S, Pawlak AP, Cho J, et al: Amphetamine's dose-dependent effects on dorsolateral striatum sensorimotor neuron firing. Behav Brain Res 244:152–161, 2013 23396149

Man KKC, Lau WCY, Coghill D, et al: Association between methylphenidate treatment and risk of seizure: a population-based, self-controlled case-series study. Lancet Child Adolesc Health 4(6):435–443, 2020 32450123

Meaden CW, Barnes S: Ketamine implicated in new onset seizure. Clin Pract Cases Emerg Med 3(4):401–404, 2019 31763599

Prasad M, Krishnan PR, Sequeira R, et al: Anticonvulsant therapy for status epilepticus. Cochrane Database Syst Rev 2014(9):CD003723, 2014 25207925

Smith SJ: EEG in the diagnosis, classification, and management of patients with epilepsy. J Neurol Neurosurg Psychiatry 76(Suppl 2):ii2–ii7, 2005 15961864

Chapter 16

Serotonin Syndrome

Memphis Diaz Garcia, M.D.
Rashi Aggarwal, M.D.

Serotonin syndrome is a result of toxic overstimulation of serotonin receptors in the CNS and the peripheral nervous system. The incidence rate of serotonin syndrome is unclear and is difficult to determine because milder forms of the condition are underreported (Boyer and Shannon 2005). Causes of serotonin syndrome may be either iatrogenic or patient-related factors. Serotonin syndrome typically occurs within the first month of a patient starting a serotonergic antidepressant, including selective serotonin reuptake inhibitors (SSRIs), monoamine oxidase inhibitors (MAOIs), tricyclic antidepressants, and selective serotonin-norepinephrine reuptake inhibitors. Starting at too high of a dose or quickly titrating up the dose of these medications as monotherapy on a treatment-naive patient may result in the precipitation of this toxidrome (Boyer 2021). More classically, iatrogenic causes have been attributed to combining these medications together or with other medications that synergistically increase the levels of serotonin in the CNS and the peripheral nervous system, especially MAOIs (Boyer and Shannon 2005). Another common drug-drug interaction includes taking the above serotonergic agents with medications that impede their metabolism by certain cytochrome oxidases in the liver (Volpi-Abadie et al. 2013).

Patient-related causes of serotonin syndrome include overdose (either accidental or intentional), although only 14%–16% of individuals who overdose on antidepressants develop serotonin syndrome (Boyer and Shannon 2005). The use of certain herbal supplements such as St. John's wort along with a serotonergic agent has been implicated in the development of this syndrome. Patients with genetic variations in the cytochrome oxidases involved in the metabolism of antidepressants, especially MAOIs, may have an increased risk of developing serotonin syndrome. A higher incidence of serotonin syndrome has been found in patients taking SSRIs who also have end-stage renal disease and are on hemodialysis, which may imply that baseline renal function is a factor in the risk for developing this toxidrome (Boyer and Shannon 2005).

Recognition and Detection

Serotonin syndrome manifests as a classic triad of altered mental status, neuromuscular abnormalities, and autonomic hyperactivity. Typical symptoms can include tremors, diarrhea, clonus, palpitations, and sweating after 24 hours of starting or increasing the dose of a serotonergic medication. In some cases, it occurs when starting a serotonergic agent within 5 weeks of discontinuing fluoxetine. In the emergency setting, serotonin syndrome can be diagnosed with the Hunter Serotonin Toxicity Criteria decision rules, which state that given a history of a serotonergic agent, the presence of any of the following suggests a positive diagnosis: 1) spontaneous clonus, 2) inducible clonus and either agitation or diaphoresis, 3) ocular clonus and either agitation or diaphoresis, 4) tremor and hyperreflexia, and 5) hypertonia with fever (temperature >38°C) and either ocular clonus or inducible clonus. An additional sixth criterion states that if none of the above criteria are present, serotonin syndrome is ruled out. The Hunter Serotonin Toxicity Criteria decision rules are 84% sensitive and 97% specific (Dunkley et al. 2003).

Culprit Medications

Medications implicated in the development of serotonin syndrome are those that have mechanisms of action that lead to the overstimulation of serotonin. The mechanisms behind the causes of serotonin syndrome can be explained by inhibition of serotonin uptake, inhibition of serotonin metabolism, increased serotonin synthesis, increased serotonin release, direct serotonin agonism, inhibition of cytochrome P450 (CYP) oxidases related to the oxidation of serotonergic agents, and decreased excretion of serotonergic agents. The following is a list of substances that function through the above mechanisms:

- Inhibition of serotonin reuptake results in decreased reuptake and increased levels of serotonin in the synaptic cleft. Substances include SSRIs, serotonin-norepinephrine reuptake inhibitors, tricyclic antidepressants, meperidine, methadone (and other opioids), dextromethorphan, St. John's wort, cocaine, and 3,4-methylenedioxymethamphetamine (MDMA).

- Inhibition of metabolism decreases the degradation of serotonin. Substances include buspirone, St. John's wort, and MAOIs.
- Increased synthesis results in increased production of serotonin released at the synapse. Substances include cocaine, amphetamines, and dietary supplements (i.e., L-tryptophan).
- Increased release is caused by substances such as mirtazapine, dextromethorphan, and MDMA.
- Direct serotonin agonists include mirtazapine, trazodone, buspirone, fentanyl, meperidine, ergotamine, and triptans.
- CYP inhibition, specifically, causes inhibition of CYP2D6 and CYP3A4 and results in increased plasma levels of certain SSRIs, including sertraline and fluoxetine, and other serotonergic agents, such as dextromethorphan. Antibiotics and antivirals such as ciprofloxacin and ritonavir also inhibit such enzymes.
- Decreased excretion can result from impaired renal function. End-stage renal disease (ESRD) has been implicated in serotonin syndrome from decreased excretion of serotonergic agents in patients with impaired renal function.

Overdose, combining multiple substances with the above mechanisms, or careless prescribing of the above medications in patients with ESRD may result in serotonin syndrome (Boyer and Shannon 2005; Volpi-Abadie et al. 2013).

Assessment

For a patient with suspected serotonin syndrome, key aspects of the history and the physical examination will guide the clinician in ruling the condition in or out. Although no laboratory studies are useful for ruling serotonin syndrome in or out, laboratory results may point to the development of complications and help rule in or out other emergencies that may have similar presentations.

Serotonin syndrome can occur in any age group. Typically, serotonin syndrome manifests within the first 24 hours of the toxic ingestion of a serotonergic agent. Therefore, the clinician must take note of the medications (prescribed and over-the-counter) that the patient may have taken before presentation, specifically those that may have serotonergic properties, and determine the time when each medication was taken. The clinician should determine whether the patient recently started any serotonergic medications or whether there were any changes, additions, or increases in medications or dosages. The clinician needs to ask about any comorbidities that may be associated with increased risk of serotonin syndrome, including, but not limited to, a history of depression, anxiety, dieting and weight loss, colds, pain syndromes, chronic pain, previous suicide attempts, and ESRD (Boyer 2021). In addition, a proper evaluation of illicit substance use (i.e., cocaine, MDMA, methamphetamine, fentanyl) or the abuse of prescription medications (i.e., phentermine, amphetamine) is important in considering the diagnosis (Boyer and Shannon 2005). Finally, the clinician should pay particular attention to symptoms related to the organ systems affected by serotonin syndrome and ask about sweats, chills, hot flashes, vision changes, tremors, restlessness, confusion, muscle tension and rigidity, nausea, vomiting, diarrhea, dry mouth, palpitations, paranoia, hypervigilance, anxiety, and akathisia (Boyer 2021; Boyer and Shannon 2005; Volpi-Abadie et al. 2013). When the patient is incapacitated, collateral information should be gathered from a reliable source because this information may affect management in severe cases.

When a patient is suspected to have serotonin syndrome, it is important to examine the patient system by system to determine the relevant findings to guide the diagnosis. The clinician should

- Pay particular attention to the systems affected by serotonin overstimulation.
- Assess vitals to determine tachycardia, hypertension, hypoxia (specifically, oxygen saturation<93%), and hyperthermia.
- Assess the mucous membranes for dryness and the pupils for mydriasis.
- Perform oculomotor testing for ocular clonus.
- Assess clonus or hypertonicity (specifically truncal rigidity because it is associated with an increased risk of respiratory failure), hyperreflexia (typically more prominent in the bilateral lower extremities), and bilateral Babinski signs.

- Check for diaphoresis and hyperactive bowel sounds.
- Complete psychiatric examination to assess increased anxiety, elements of cognition, disorientation, agitation, and thought content for any hypervigilance or paranoid ideations (Boyer 2021; Volpi-Abadie et al. 2013).

No laboratory tests are needed to make a diagnosis of serotonin syndrome, nor is there any specific laboratory test that directly rules this toxidrome in or out (Boyer 2021). Note that not only are serotonin levels not readily available in most hospital laboratories, but also the level of serotonin in the blood is not correlated with the severity of the presentation (Volpi-Abadie et al. 2013). However, some laboratory tests and other studies may be of value in the emergent presentation of a patient with serotonin syndrome.

A complete blood count typically shows leukocytosis. Thrombocytopenia, elevated prothrombin time, and activated partial thromboplastin time may be seen in severe cases of serotonin syndrome leading to disseminated intravascular coagulation (Boral et al. 2016). Basic metabolic panels can show elevated creatinine suggestive of acute kidney injury or failure related to complications from rhabdomyolysis and myoglobinuria (Boyer and Shannon 2005). Elevated creatinine also may be related to a history of ESRD, which may be seen with additional electrolyte abnormalities in the basic metabolic panel (hyperkalemia, hyperphosphatemia). Urinalysis provides more information on myoglobinuria, and elevated creatine kinase suggests rhabdomyolysis from prolonged sustained leaden paralysis from hypertonia (Boyer and Shannon 2005). Basic metabolic panel and blood gas analysis may show metabolic acidosis because of lactic acidosis in relation to severe hypertonia. Blood gases with further clinical assessment may also point to the severe complication of acute respiratory distress syndrome (Boyer 2021; Edriss 2014). Finally, urine toxicology may provide information on exposure to substances that may be contributing to the presentation of serotonin syndrome (i.e., amphetamines, opioids) (Boyer 2021; Volpi-Abadie et al. 2013). Of note, thyrotoxicosis should be ruled out, and therefore, thyroid function tests may be beneficial as well (Boyer 2021; Cooper 2003).

In addition to the presentation of sinus tachycardia on an electrocardiogram in serotonin syndrome, there have been case reports of patients developing atrial fibrillation 6 hours after ingestion of a serotonergic agent. T-wave flattening, T-wave inversions, and ventricular tachycardia also have been reported (Dudum et al. 2018), which raises concern for patients with conditions that already predispose them to arrhythmias.

It is important to differentiate between serotonin syndrome and other toxidromes that may have a similar presentation. These toxidromes include neuroleptic malignant syndrome (NMS), malignant hyperthermia, anticholinergic toxicity, and thyrotoxicosis (Boyer 2021; Volpi-Abadie et al. 2013). NMS is a toxidrome related to exposure to dopamine antagonists that poses a challenge in differentiating it from serotonin syndrome because patients also present with autonomic dysfunction, neuromuscular changes, and alterations in mental status. In addition, patients presenting with either NMS or serotonin syndrome may be taking both a serotonergic agent and a neuroleptic agent (Tse et al. 2015). Unlike serotonin syndrome, NMS results in neuromuscular hypoactivity, specifically bradyreflexia, rather than hyperreflexia and inducible clonus. The timeline is also different, with symptoms typically occurring days to weeks after exposure to a neuroleptic rather than within 24 hours in the case of serotonin syndrome (Tse et al. 2015; Volpi-Abadie et al. 2013). Malignant hyperthermia is a toxidrome related to exposure to inhaled anesthetics and depolarizing muscle relaxants that results in skin mottling, cyanosis, and hyporeflexia in addition to muscle rigidity, occurring minutes to hours after exposure. Anticholinergic toxicity, as the name implies, is associated with toxic exposure to anticholinergics, which results in urinary retention, *decreased* bowel sounds, dry skin, erythema, and *normal* muscle tone and reflexes in addition to hyperthermia (Volpi-Abadie et al. 2013). Thyrotoxicosis is associated with exposure to significant levels of the thyroid hormone, through either exogenous or endogenous sources, resulting in hyperthermia, tremors, tachycardia, diaphoresis, and anxiety, but it is found in patients who have elevated thyroid hormone levels; muscle rigidity is not a typical finding (Cooper 2003).

Management

It is paramount to *immediately* discontinue the offending agents and to start conservative measures to manage vitals and temperature. These measures can include cooling blankets, intravenous hydration, and benzodiazepines. Specifically, diazepam has been noted to help in the management of mild hypertension, tachycardia, and mild fevers. Diazepam also helps in the management of acute agitation in the setting of serotonin syndrome (Volpi-Abadie et al. 2013). Diazepam may be administered in 5- to 10-mg IV doses, given every 8–10 minutes, titrated for the desired effects. Alternatively, 2- to 4-mg IV lorazepam can be administered every 8–10 minutes as needed (Boyer 2021).

After being stabilized, the patient should be observed for at least 6 hours to ensure that there are no further complications. If the patient has persistent symptoms, starting the patient on serotonin antagonists, specifically cyproheptadine, is recommended. Cyproheptadine has a significant affinity for the serotonin 2A receptor, thereby effectively antagonizing the neurochemical culprit behind serotonin syndrome (Boyer and Shannon 2005). Typically, cyproheptadine is given orally at an initial dose of 12 mg, followed by an additional 2 mg every 2 hours until clinical response is reached. Afterward, it is dosed at 4–8 mg every 6 hours as needed, with a maximum dosage of 32 mg per 24 hours (Sun-Edelstein et al. 2008). Note that there are important contraindications for the use of this medication, including oversedation and hypotension in elderly adults and excitation in pediatric populations; it is also contraindicated for patients with cardiovascular disease, thyroid dysfunction, asthma, and glaucoma because cyproheptadine can worsen these conditions (A-S Medication Solutions 2022). Patients with moderate cases of serotonin syndrome require admission for cardiac monitoring and further observation. Severe presentations may include severe hyperthermia (temperatures >41.1°C), severe hemodynamic instability, spontaneous and sustained clonus, severe muscle rigidity, and delirium. Once patients have reached this stage in their presentation, cyproheptadine has not been shown to provide any additional benefit. Patients with severe presentations may need to be admitted to an intensive care unit for a higher level of care and require intubation and sedation.

Severe hypertension and tachycardia are managed with short-acting antihypertensive agents, including esmolol and nitroprusside. Longer-acting agents, such as propranolol, are avoided because they can cause severe hypotension in those who are hemodynamically unstable. Esmolol and nitroprusside also do not result in significant masking of tachycardia, which is important because heart rate is used as a marker of treatment response. Sedation and paralysis should be achieved with a nondepolarizing agent, such as vecuronium. Succinyl-choline and other depolarizing muscle relaxants should be avoided as paralyzing agents because they are associated with worsening hyperkalemia and rhabdomyolysis (Scotton et al. 2019; Volpi-Abadie et al. 2013).

Follow-Up Management

Fortunately, serotonin syndrome has a very favorable prognosis if treatment is provided, with cases of complete resolution of symptoms without long-term effects (Mason et al. 2000). A careful review of medications is warranted after the patient has been stabilized. If two serotonergic agents are used together, they should be used with caution (Volpi-Abadie et al. 2013). Medications with similar mechanisms of action should be discontinued, or treatment should be simplified by using a medication that targets multiple desired effects. Unfortunately, the development of serotonin syndrome cannot be predicted because a vast number of medications have serotonergic properties, and the list continues to grow.

Conclusion

In general, serotonin syndrome is a toxidrome that has significant relevance in psychiatric, primary medical, and emergency medical practice with the increasing use of antidepressants in the United States. Given the increasing use of serotonergic agents, it is important to evaluate and detect symptoms suspicious of serotonin syndrome so that timely and appropriate management can be provided. It is important to weigh the risks and benefits of using these medications with patients before making any final medication changes. Screening at every visit or when medications are changed or added may be beneficial in preventing further complications.

Key Points

Serotonin syndrome is characterized by a triad of altered mental status, neuromuscular abnormalities, and autonomic hyperactivity, which can range from mild to severe.

Causes of serotonin syndrome include iatrogenic and non-iatrogenic factors that lead to serotonergic overstimulation.

The Hunter Serotonin Toxicity Criteria decision rules are a reliable set of criteria for determining the diagnosis.

Other toxidromes such as neuroleptic malignant syndrome, malignant hyperthermia, and anticholinergic toxicity, which may have a presentation similar to serotonin syndrome, should be ruled out.

Management of serotonin syndrome includes discontinuation of the offending agent, stabilizing vitals, and preventing worsening of rigidity and hyperthermia; cyproheptadine is reserved for mild to moderate cases, whereas severe cases require intensive care unit management and intravenous antihypertensive medications.

References

A-S Medication Solutions: CYPROHEPTADINE HYDROCHLORIDE- cyproheptadine hydrochloride tablet. FDALabel, October 5, 2022. Available at: https://nctr-crs.fda.gov/fdalabel/services/spl/set-ids/0e43e99b-2e0b-4f55-b93a-a6908634880d/spl-doc?hl=cyproheptadine. Accessed November 2, 2022.

Boral BM, Williams DJ, Boral LI: Disseminated intravascular coagulation. Am J Clin Pathol 146(6):670–680, 2016 28013226

Boyer EW: Serotonin syndrome (serotonin toxicity). UpToDate, April 5, 2021. Available at: https://www.uptodate.com/contents/serotonin-syndrome-serotonin-toxicity. Accessed July 10, 2022.

Boyer EW, Shannon M: The serotonin syndrome. N Engl J Med 352(11):1112–1120, 2005 15784664

Cooper DS: Hyperthyroidism. Lancet 362(9382):459–468, 2003 12927435

Dudum R, Aslam MI, Madrazo J: Serotonin syndrome masquerading as ventricular tachycardia storm. Am J Med 131(12):e498–e499, 2018 30077498

Dunkley EJC, Isbister GK, Sibbritt D, et al: The Hunter Serotonin Toxicity Criteria: simple and accurate diagnostic decision rules for serotonin toxicity. QJM 96(9):635–642, 2003 12925718

Edriss H: Acute respiratory distress syndrome, metabolic acidosis, and respiratory acidosis associated with citalopram overdose. The Southwest Respiratory and Critical Care Chronicles 2(5):24, 2014

Mason PJ, Morris VA, Balczak TJ: Serotonin syndrome: presentation of 2 cases and review of the literature. Medicine (Baltimore) 79(4):201–209, 2000 10941349

Scotton WJ, Hill LJ, Williams AC, Barnes NM: Serotonin syndrome: pathophysiology, clinical features, management, and potential future directions. Int J Tryptophan Res 12:1178646919873925, 2019 31523132

Sun-Edelstein C, Tepper SJ, Shapiro RE: Drug-induced serotonin syndrome: a review. Expert Opin Drug Saf 7(5):587–596, 2008 18759711

Tse L, Barr AM, Scarapicchia V, Vila-Rodriguez F: Neuroleptic malignant syndrome: a review from a clinically oriented perspective. Curr Neuropharmacol 13(3):395–406, 2015 26411967

Volpi-Abadie J, Kaye AM, Kaye AD: Serotonin syndrome. Ochsner J 13(4):533–540, 2013 24358002

Chapter 17

Substances With Addictive Potential and Psychotropic Medications

Peter J. Na, M.D., M.P.H.
Sanya Virani, M.D., M.P.H.
Oluwole Jegede, M.D., M.P.H.
Adrienne Hicks, M.D., Ph.D.
Sivabalaji Kaliamurthy, M.D.
Aaron Wolfgang, M.D.
Ellen L. Edens, M.D.

Use of addictive drugs, whether prescribed or non-prescribed, frequently co-occurs and complicates pharmacological management of psychiatric conditions. Additionally, nonprescribed drugs are unregulated and often adulterated with other unknown substances, requiring a broad workup. We describe the most common and significant interactions between addictive drugs (including ethanol and nicotine but excluding opioids and benzodiazepines, which are discussed in Chapter 4, "Benzodiazepines in Combination With Opioids: Therapeutic Benefit Versus Fatal Overdose") and psychotropic medications to assist clinically sound psychopharmacological treatment.

The views expressed herein are those of the authors and do not reflect the views or policy of the U.S. Government, Department of Defense, Department of Veterans Affairs, U.S. Army, or Brooke Army Medical Center.

Culprit Substances and Medications

Ethanol

Recognition and Detection

Ethanol consumption causes direct interactions with many psychotropic medications, including antidepressants, anxiolytics, and antipsychotics. Chronic ingestion of alcohol induces certain hepatic enzymes, resulting in enhanced medication elimination and diminished therapeutic effects.

The primary concerns when combining ethanol with antidepressants, especially tricyclic antidepressants (TCAs), include oversedation and altered antidepressant metabolism, leading to increased risk of adverse medication events. For example, concurrent amitriptyline and ethanol use is associated with a marked increase in body sway, decreased manual dexterity, and decreased short-term memory (Chan and Anderson 2014).

When selective serotonin and serotonin-norepinephrine reuptake inhibitors are combined with ethanol, several interactions have been seen. Venlafaxine, escitalopram, and sertraline increase the risk of gastrointestinal or other bleeding as a result of antiplatelet effects augmented by inhibition of platelet serotonin uptake. Duloxetine, when combined with ethanol, may lead to hypotension, including orthostasis, and abrupt cessation of ethanol use in those taking bupropion may increase risk of seizures (ethanol withdrawal or excessive use may lower seizure threshold) (Chan and Anderson 2014).

Ethanol alters first-pass metabolism of amitriptyline in the liver, resulting in increased amitriptyline levels in the blood and leading to several potential interactions. Additionally, alcohol-induced liver disease may further impair amitriptyline breakdown and result in increased levels of active medication in the body (i.e., increased bioavailability). High amitriptyline levels, in turn, can lead to convulsions and disturbances in heart rhythm.

People prescribed monoamine oxidase inhibitors (MAOIs) are advised to adhere to a low-tyramine diet because elevated tyramine can lead to a potentially life-threatening hypertensive crisis. All ethanol-containing beverages have been fermented, and some have high levels of tyramine. Thus, caution is advised when consuming ethanol, especially beverages produced using a nonstandard fermentation process.

Antipsychotic medications combined with ethanol may potentiate the risk of CNS and respiratory depression as well as psychomotor impairment. Other CNS depressants, including benzodiazepines, barbiturates, and nonbenzodiazepine sedative-hypnotics, have a synergistic effect when combined with alcohol, potentiating the likelihood for dangerous and even lethal consequences, a major emergency with rapid onset of dizziness, stumbling, loss of sphincter control, memory loss, and potential death.

Stimulants can mask the effects of ethanol, make it difficult for people to gauge their level of intoxication, and result in overconsumption and greater intoxication. Ethanol toxicity is evidenced by impaired coordination, impaired judgment, blackout, passing out, and potential death. Experts recommend avoiding the intake of methylphenidate in the form of extended-release capsules or orally disintegrating tablets in combination with ethanol because of a phenomenon known as *dose dumping* that may lead to stimulant toxicity (Childress et al. 2019). Patients who have stimulant toxicity present with dry mouth, hyperthermia, dilated pupils, tachypnea, increased alertness and energy, and sometimes chest pain and palpitations.

Disulfiram, an FDA-approved treatment for alcohol use disorder, is used for the aversive effect it causes when combined with ethanol. The disulfiram-ethanol reaction leads to increased levels of serum acetaldehyde, causing diaphoresis, palpitations, facial flushing, nausea, vertigo, hypotension, and tachycardia.

Assessment

Patients will usually present with sedation or respiratory depression and sometimes seizures or hypertensive crises and will less often present with increased bleeding or arrhythmias. Routine laboratory work such as blood ethanol level must be obtained if ethanol intoxication is among the differential diagnoses. Ethyl glucuronide and ethyl sulfate are direct biomarkers of ethanol and can be detected in urine for up to 5 days.

Management

When an ethanol-medication interaction is suspected, it is critical to evaluate and maintain airway and breathing, and adequate oxygenation and ventilation should be ensured.

Proper documentation of other medications and patterns of ethanol consumption, especially over time, will assist clinical decision-making. Before starting psychopharmacological therapy, it is essential for providers to screen for the presence of at-risk ethanol consumption, evaluate the presence of an alcohol use disorder, and explain the potential harms of combining ethanol with psychotropic medication.

Stimulants

Recognition and Detection

Stimulants are a class of substances that include plant alkaloid derivatives such as cocaine, ephedra, and khat and synthetic compounds such as amphetamines. These substances are important for their pharmacological and clinical applications, potential for addiction, induction of acute behavioral and physiological symptoms in withdrawal and overdose states, and potential fatality in toxic states.

Stimulants may enhance the serotonergic effects of selective serotonin and serotonin-norepinephrine reuptake inhibitors and result in potentially fatal serotonin syndrome (Gallelli et al. 2017). Bupropion lowers the seizure threshold and may significantly increase the risk of seizures in patients taking stimulants. A few cases of serotonin syndrome also have been reported when bupropion was combined with amphetamines (Munhoz 2004; Thorpe et al. 2010).

TCAs may potentiate the cardiovascular effects of stimulants, particularly in patients with cardiovascular comorbidity, such as arrhythmias, orthostasis, and congestive heart failure. Serotonin syndrome is also a risk when combining TCAs and stimulants.

All MAOIs, including isocarboxazid, tranylcypromine, phenelzine, and selegiline, should be avoided in patients taking stimulants. MAOI and stimulant interaction results in a surge and overload of monoamine activity, which may lead to hypertensive crisis, hyperthermia, seizures, and, potentially, intracranial hemorrhage.

Stimulants combined with mood stabilizers may increase the risk of serotonin syndrome, alter the metabolism of the mood stabilizer, or increase the risk for seizures. Specifically, combining lithium with stimulants may enhance the serotonergic effects of lithium, resulting in serotonin syndrome. In patients with a seizure disorder treated with an antiepileptic, stimulants may decrease seizure threshold and potentially interfere with seizure pharmacotherapy.

β-Adrenergic-blocking agents are sometimes used in psychiatric disorders. When they are combined with cocaine or other stimulants, unopposed and excessive stimulation of α-adrenergic receptors may occur, resulting in severe vasoconstriction, hypertension, and cardiac arrhythmias (Richards et al. 2017).

Co-use of nonprescribed and prescribed stimulant medication can result in sympathetic overactivation, manifesting as hypertensive crisis, seizure, cardiac arrhythmias, cardiovascular collapse, and death. There is an increased risk of serotonin syndrome in patients prescribed amphetamines who also use cocaine (Devlin and Henry 2008; Silins et al. 2007).

Assessment

Patients may present with signs and symptoms of hypertensive crisis, serotonergic or cardiovascular toxicity, seizures, or psychosis. The assessment of patients will follow the presenting symptoms. The diagnosis of serotonin syndrome is made clinically, with a thorough medication history and physical and neurological examination. The most frequently used diagnostic standard is the Hunter Serotonin Toxicity Criteria, a six-item scale that asks about toxicity symptoms in the presence of a serotonergic agent (Werneke et al. 2020). Although not confirmatory, initial laboratory investigations are necessary to determine differential diagnoses and to monitor for potential complications and response to treatment. All positive amphetamine screens should be followed by confirmation testing, such as gas chromatography–mass spectrometry. Methylphenidate, which is structurally dissimilar to amphetamines, will not be detected by a routine amphetamine screen, and a separate test must be ordered. Emerging synthetic cathinones are not included on regular urine drug screen panels; therefore, clinicians must continue to rely on clinical presentation and history when managing patients who are taking stimulants.

Management

The mainstay of treatment is prevention of life-threatening catecholaminergic and serotonin toxicity by avoiding combinations of drugs as described earlier in the "Recognition and Detection" section in patients who use stimulants, have a stimulant use disorder, or are being prescribed amphetamines. It is recommended that prescribed stimulants be discontinued at least 2 weeks before the initiation of an MAOI. Serotonin syndrome must be treated as a medical emergency. Definitive management consists of discontinuation of the offending drugs, supportive care, sedation, and administration of serotonergic antagonists such as cyproheptadine.

Cannabinoids

Recognition and Detection

Cannabinoid use, including both delta-9-tetrahydrocannabinol (Δ-9-THC) and cannabidiol (CBD), is gaining widespread acceptance in the United States, and intoxication and drug-medication interactions can easily be overlooked or disregarded during medical emergencies. Chemicals found in the cannabis plant and synthetic cannabinoids have a strong association with emergence of psychotic symptoms and even aggressive and/or violent behavior. Some hybrid strains have a very high percentage of Δ-9-THC, the primary psychoactive cannabinoid, causing harmful effects when combined with certain medications, especially during cannabis intoxication.

Caution is advised with co-use of psychotropics that are substrates of cytochromes affected by cannabis itself or cannabis inhalation; Δ-9-THC inhibits cytochrome P450 2C9 (CYP2C9) and CYP3A4, CBD inhibits CYP2C19 and CYP3A4, and cannabis inhalation inhibits CYP1A1 and CYP1A2 (Rong et al. 2018). For example, when coadministered with venlafaxine, cannabis can intensify drowsiness and sedation and exacerbate hypertension and tachycardia, which are known side effects of venlafaxine. Cannabis may worsen symptoms of irritability, nervousness, and jitteriness when used with fluoxetine and, like when it is combined with venlafaxine, may exacerbate sedation, hypertension, and tachycardia when used with TCAs. It has been reported that bupropion exacerbates cannabis withdrawal (e.g., irritability, restlessness, depression, insomnia) (Brezing and Levin 2018).

Cannabis may exacerbate the tachycardia and cardiovascular side effects known to occur with stimulant use. Barbiturates and both benzodiazepine and nonbenzodiazepine sedative-hypnotics should be avoided during acute cannabis intoxication to avoid additive effects of sedation (Johnstone et al. 1975). Cannabis may also potentiate sedation and tachycardia if taken with antihistamines, such as diphenhydramine.

Assessment

Signs and symptoms of cannabis intoxication vary from mild sedation to psychosis. Because synthetic cannabinoids will not show up in a routine urine drug screen, obtaining a thorough history is essential. Clinicians who suspect synthetic cannabinoid use will need to consult laboratory medicine to order the correct test capable of detection. Patients should be monitored and managed according to symptom severity while clinicians work up differential diagnoses. An assessment of a cannabis use disorder is critical.

Management

Cardiac symptoms, most commonly tachycardia and hypertension, require close monitoring because they are side effects of many psychotropic medications and of acute cannabis intoxication. Other known side effects, such as psychosis, agitation, sedation, bleeding, and hyperglycemia, also should be monitored in patients who use cannabinoid products. The perception that cannabis use is largely safe and has limited risks is increasing. An emergency setting is a critical time to provide individually tailored education on the real and perceived risks of cannabis as well as to deliver a brief intervention for people prescribed psychotropic medications who also use cannabis daily and/or heavily.

Nicotine and Cigarette Smoking

Recognition and Detection

Nicotine-related medication interactions are pharmacodynamic in nature and are uncommon. However, clinicians should monitor for emergent hypertension in patients taking bupropion and nicotine replacement therapy (U.S. Food and Drug Administration 2011). Polycyclic aromatic hydrocarbons, a by-product of cigarette smoking, lead to pharmacokinetic interactions by induction of hepatic CYP enzymes (Desai et al. 2001). The primary concern related to cigarette smoking is when smoking levels change (e.g., during smoking cessation or initiation). Polycyclic aromatic hydrocarbons are a potent inducer of CYP1A2 and CYP2B6, enzymes that metabolize several clinically important psychotropic medications. Specifically, CYP1A2 metabolizes several antidepressants (amitriptyline, imipramine, duloxetine, fluvoxamine) and antipsychotics (clozapine, haloperidol, olanzapine), whereas CYP2B6 is involved in metabolism of bupropion and methadone (Desai et al. 2001; Oliveira et al. 2017; Zevin and Benowitz 1999). The effect of smoking on hepatic enzymes is not related to the nicotine component of tobacco, and nicotine replacement therapy does not influence CYP activity.

Therefore, when people stop cigarette smoking by choice or during a hospitalization, medication levels can increase, resulting in toxicity. Particular caution is advised when managing a patient prescribed clozapine. Clozapine toxicity, which can be lethal, is associated with hyperthermia, alterations in consciousness, seizures, cardiac arrhythmias, excessive mucus production in bronchi, hypersalivation, miosis, blood dyscrasias, pancreatitis, and hepatitis.

Signs of antidepressant toxicity can include anxiety, irritability, nausea, somnolence, insomnia, and tremors. Extrapyramidal side effects should be monitored in patients prescribed antipsychotics.

Additionally, cigarette smoke exerts an indirect effect on lithium metabolism by altering caffeine metabolism (Frigerio et al. 2021). Clinicians should check lithium levels if clinical concerns arise. Cigarette smoke also increases clearance of propranolol from the body, rendering it less effective (Zevin and Benowitz 1999). Bradycardia may manifest as a result of smoking cessation and rapid increase in serum β-blocker levels.

No currently available evidence suggests that vapors produced by electronic nicotine delivery systems significantly affect the metabolism of psychotropic medications. This area of research is still nascent.

Assessment

The most critical presentation related to smoking cessation and psychotropic medication is clozapine toxicity. If a patient presents with history and symptoms of clozapine toxicity (e.g., hyperthermia, alterations in consciousness, seizures, cardiac arrhythmias, excessive mucus production in bronchi, hypersalivation, miosis, blood dyscrasias, pancreatitis, hepatitis), then clozapine and norclozapine levels should be obtained.

Management

Management of clozapine toxicity is generally limited to symptomatic therapy, such as airway management, intravenous fluids for hypotension, and monitoring. All people who smoke nicotine should be encouraged to stop and be supported during quit attempts. Side effects and potential medication toxicity can be minimized through careful medication dose adjustment, especially when a patient is attempting to stop nicotine use.

Psychedelics

Recognition and Detection

The three most used psychedelics globally are 3,4-methylenedioxymethamphetamine (MDMA; commonly referred to as ecstasy), lysergic acid diethylamide (LSD, or acid), and psilocybin (magic mushrooms). Although considered relatively safe, psychedelics may pose a risk when combined with other psychiatric medications or nonprescribed substances.

Both bupropion and MDMA are substrates and inhibitors of CYP2D6, leading to increased serum concentrations of each. Co-use of MDMA and bupropion, therefore, lowers the seizure threshold and increases the risk of seizures (Cohen et al. 2021).

TCAs are also substrates of CYP2D6. As with bupropion, the combination of MDMA and TCAs increases the concentrations of both, which elevates the risk of cardiotoxicity, arrhythmias, and sudden cardiac death.

The combination of MAOIs and MDMA may precipitate a potentially lethal serotonin syndrome, although so-called classic psychedelics, including LSD and psilocybin, do not (Bonson and Murphy 1996). The combination of a classic psychedelic and lithium may potentiate the effects of the psychedelic and also may increase the risk of seizures (Nayak et al. 2021).

Assessment

Serotonin syndrome, syndrome of inappropriate antidiuretic hormone, hyponatremia, heatstroke, cardiotoxicity, and seizures are the most urgent conditions to assess (Cohen et al. 2021; Nayak et al. 2021). The necessary workup includes a complete blood count, a comprehensive metabolic panel, hepatic function tests, creatine phosphokinase levels, coagulation studies, a urinalysis, a urine drug screen, and an electrocardiogram.

Management

Individuals seeking acute care related to psychedelic use most often will be treated in an emergency setting with medical admission as indicated. Serotonergic agents should be discontinued, and supportive care should be provided to correct vital signs. Benzodiazepines may be considered to treat anxiety, agitation, or seizures. Cyproheptadine may be used to reverse the effects of a coadministered serotonergic medication or potentially the psychedelic itself.

Follow-Up Management

In most cases, acute interaction should prompt holding or discontinuing the prescribed psychotropic medication. Once acute issues are resolved, however, a clinical decision must be made to reinitiate the medication, transition to an alternative medication with less safety risk, or discontinue pharmacological treatment altogether. Although a conscientious substance use evaluation is essential at this juncture, the presence of an active substance use disorder is rarely, if ever, an absolute contraindication to continuing treatment for co-occurring psychiatric conditions. Rather, clinical decision-making should be grounded in patient-centered, clear communication about the risks, benefits, and monitoring plan of various options. If a substance use disorder is diagnosed, evidence-based treatment should be initiated (Department of Veterans Affairs and Department of Defense 2021). For at-risk substance use, brief interventions delivered in emergency settings can have a powerful effect on future behaviors (Hawk and D'Onofrio 2018).

Conclusion

Potentially addictive substances, prescribed or nonprescribed, have variable interactions with psychotropic medications ranging from irritability to cardiotoxicity. Nonprescribed substances have added concern given their unregulated and often adulterated content. Given the increase in recreational substance use in the United States and the high prevalence of co-occurring psychiatric disorders in individuals who have substance use disorders, clinicians should be familiar with potentially harmful addictive substance–psychotropic medication interactions.

Key Points

Addictive drugs can negatively interact with psychotropic medications.

Ethanol may cause excessive sedation and respiratory depression.

Stimulants may cause psychosis, serotonin syndrome, or hypertensive crisis.

Cannabinoids are associated with psychosis and tachycardia and, when combined with CNS depressants, may cause excessive sedation.

Nicotine cessation or initiation may affect psychotropic blood levels, resulting in critical conditions such as clozapine toxicity.

3,4-Methylenedioxymethamphetamine (MDMA) may lead to seizures when coadministered with bupropion, cardiotoxicity when combined with tricyclic antidepressants, and serotonin syndrome when used with monoamine oxidase inhibitors.

Use of addictive drugs is not an absolute contraindication to pharmacological treatment of co-occurring psychiatric conditions. Guideline-concordant care requires a thorough substance use evaluation with provision of brief interventions or initiation of treatment as indicated.

References

Bonson KR, Murphy DL: Alterations in responses to LSD in humans associated with chronic administration of tricyclic antidepressants, monoamine oxidase inhibitors or lithium. Behav Brain Res 73(1–2):229–233, 1996 8788508

Brezing CA, Levin FR: The current state of pharmacological treatments for cannabis use disorder and withdrawal. Neuropsychopharmacology 43(1):173–194, 2018 28875989

Chan LN, Anderson GD: Pharmacokinetic and pharmacodynamic drug interactions with ethanol (alcohol). Clin Pharmacokinet 53(12):1115–1136, 2014 25267448

Childress AC, Komolova M, Sallee FR: An update on the pharmacokinetic considerations in the treatment of ADHD with long-acting methylphenidate and amphetamine formulations. Expert Opin Drug Metab Toxicol 15(11):937–974, 2019 31581854

Cohen IV, Makunts T, Abagyan R, Thomas K: Concomitant drugs associated with increased mortality for MDMA users reported in a drug safety surveillance database. Sci Rep 11(1):5997, 2021 33727616

Department of Veterans Affairs and Department of Defense: VA/DoD clinical practice guideline for the management of substance use disorders. 2021. Available at: www.healthquality.va.gov/guidelines/MH/sud/VADoDSUDCPG.pdf. Accessed October 1, 2021.

Desai HD, Seabolt J, Jann MW: Smoking in patients receiving psychotropic medications: a pharmacokinetic perspective. CNS Drugs 15(6):469–494, 2001 11524025

Devlin RJ, Henry JA: Clinical review: major consequences of illicit drug consumption. Crit Care 12(1):202, 2008 18279535

Frigerio S, Strawbridge R, Young AH: The impact of caffeine consumption on clinical symptoms in patients with bipolar disorder: a systematic review. Bipolar Disord 23(3):241–251, 2021 32949106

Gallelli L, Gratteri S, Siniscalchi A, et al: Drug-drug interactions in cocaine-users and their clinical implications. Curr Drug Abuse Rev 10(1):25–30, 2017 29185916

Hawk K, D'Onofrio G: Emergency department screening and interventions for substance use disorders. Addict Sci Clin Pract 13(1):18, 2018 30078375

Johnstone RE, Lief PL, Kulp RA, Smith TC: Combination of delta9-tetrahydrocannabinol with oxymorphone or pentobarbital: effects on ventilatory control and cardiovascular dynamics. Anesthesiology 42(6):674–684, 1975 48348

Munhoz RP: Serotonin syndrome induced by a combination of bupropion and SSRIs. Clin Neuropharmacol 27(5):219–222, 2004 15602102

Nayak SM, Gukasyan N, Barrett FS, et al: Classic psychedelic co-administration with lithium, but not lamotrigine, is associated with seizures: an analysis of online psychedelic experience reports. Pharmacopsychiatry 54(5):240–245, 2021 34348413

Oliveira P, Ribeiro J, Donato H, Madeira N: Smoking and antidepressants pharmacokinetics: a systematic review. Ann Gen Psychiatry 16:17, 2017 28286537

Richards JR, Hollander JE, Ramoska EA, et al: β-blockers, cocaine, and the unopposed α-stimulation phenomenon. J Cardiovasc Pharmacol Ther 22(3):239–249, 2017 28399647

Rong C, Carmona NE, Lee YL, et al: Drug-drug interactions as a result of co-administering Δ^9-THC and CBD with other psychotropic agents. Expert Opin Drug Saf 17(1):51–54, 2018 29082802

Silins E, Copeland J, Dillon P: Qualitative review of serotonin syndrome, ecstasy (MDMA) and the use of other serotonergic substances: hierarchy of risk. Aust N Z J Psychiatry 41(8):649–655, 2007 17620161

Thorpe EL, Pizon AF, Lynch MJ, Boyer J: Bupropion induced serotonin syndrome: a case report. J Med Toxicol 6(2):168–171, 2010 20238197

U.S. Food and Drug Administration: Zyban: prescribing information. 2011. Available at: www.accessdata.fda.gov/drugsatfda_docs/label/2011/020711s026lbl.pdf. Accessed October 1, 2021.

Werneke U, Truedson-Martiniussen P, Wikström H, Ott M: Serotonin syndrome: a clinical review of current controversies. J Integr Neurosci 19(4):719–727, 2020 33378846

Zevin S, Benowitz NL: Drug interactions with tobacco smoking: an update. Clin Pharmacokinet 36(6):425–438, 1999 10427467

Chapter 18

Tardive Dyskinesia

Michael D. Jibson, M.D., Ph.D.

Tardive dyskinesia (TD; literally translating to "late bad movements") is a motor disorder consisting of involuntary choreiform (i.e., irregular, spasmodic) or athetoid (i.e., slow, writhing) movements of the face, trunk, or limbs. It is most often, although not exclusively, associated with long-term use of antipsychotic medications, generally developing after months or years of treatment. The symptoms are both stigmatizing and potentially disabling, in extreme cases interfering with grooming, hygiene, mobility, and even eating.

The pathophysiology of TD is not well understood, and most proposed mechanisms are based on animal models rather than clinical studies. A role for dopamine is well established on the basis of the propensity of dopamine antagonists and partial agonists to cause symptoms and, conversely, the dopamine-depleting actions of drugs known to treat those symptoms. Within that framework, the most commonly cited mechanism involves excess blockade of dopamine D_2 receptors compared with D_1 receptors in the basal ganglia. D_1 receptors function primarily to activate striatal pathways that are opposed by D_2-mediated neurons; hence, drugs with greater D_2 blockade (e.g., haloperidol) tend to leave D_1-controlled systems excessively activated, whereas drugs with greater D_1 binding (e.g., clozapine) restrict that activity. Output from this pathway is further mediated by GABAergic, glutamatergic, and cholinergic neurons, each of which may play a role in both the production and the treatment of abnormal movements. This model has the merit of accounting for the differences in TD risk between older and newer antipsychotic drugs, but convincing clinical evidence for it has been sparse, and trials of numerous agents that modulate these additional pathways have not yielded appreciable benefits.

The prevalence of the disorder has been the subject of much debate. In the era of first-generation antipsychotics

(FGAs), incident rates of about 5% per year of exposure were typically cited, requiring prescribers to make special mention of the risk during routine procedures of informed consent. In the first decade of second-generation antipsychotics (SGAs), their risk was thought to be dramatically lower than that of FGAs, and regular disclosure to patients of this potential adverse effect became less common. More recent studies have shown that the differences are less dramatic than initially suggested, with one large meta-analysis placing the annual incidence of TD at 6.5% for FGAs and 2.6% for SGAs (Carbon et al. 2018). Because many patients take these medications for years or even decades, the overall prevalence of TD that accrues has been estimated at 7% for patients exposed exclusively to SGAs, 23% for patients currently taking SGAs but previously treated with FGAs, and 30% for those taking primarily FGAs over their entire course of treatment (Carbon et al. 2017). These numbers make clear that patients face significant risk of TD when prescribed antipsychotics of any kind over an extended period but support the use of SGAs in preference to FGAs to mitigate that risk.

Concerns about nonmodifiable factors, such as age and race, have similarly evolved. Early studies involving mostly FGAs reported dramatically higher risk in older individuals, irrespective of the disorder being treated, noting incidence rates as high as 20% per year of exposure for patients older than 65 years (Jeste et al. 1995). For older patients (mean age=78 years) never previously exposed to antipsychotics, one prospective study found an annual TD incidence of 5.7% with SGAs, about twice that in younger patients (Woerner et al. 2011).

Asians and Black Americans have similarly been reported to bear higher risk (Tarsy and Baldessarini 2006). Some studies, however, have shown different patterns across age and racial groups. Carbon and colleagues (2017), for example, found no differences across age groups and a twofold lower incidence among Asians in their meta-analysis.

Other risk factors are less contributory but are occasionally noted. Women tend to have higher rates of TD than do men. Those with mood disorders typically have higher rates of all types of movement disorders, including TD, than do patients with schizophrenia. Patients with significant extrapyramidal side effects may carry elevated risk. Exposure to anticholinergic drugs has been cited as a potential risk factor, but this relationship appears to be a consequence of selective anticholinergic use in patients with high rates of extrapyramidal side effects rather than a direct effect of the drugs.

For patients in all groups, duration of exposure to high-risk medication is critical, with risk beginning in as little as 1 month of treatment and increasing without plateau over years of use. The effect of drug dose is less clear. Although it is generally assumed that higher doses carry greater risk, studies have shown comparable rates of the disorder in patients maintained on high and low levels of antipsychotics (Tarsy and Baldessarini 2006).

Movement disorders such as TD were described in patients with schizophrenia before the advent of antipsychotic medications, albeit at a lower frequency and severity than among medication-exposed patients. Because nearly all cases of schizophrenia are now treated with antipsychotics, little effort is made to differentiate between cases related to the diagnosis and those caused by the drugs. Tics in Tourette's disorder involve various involuntary movements, some of which may be confused with TD, especially those involving the lips, tongue, or face. The primary differentiating factors are the underlying drive experienced with tics and their sudden, brief expression, as opposed to the longer duration and more writhing quality of TD. Individuals with autism often display repetitive movements, such as rocking or atypical hand movements. Differentiation of the disorders is usually based on a long-standing diagnosis of autism and the somewhat different appearance of the movements. TD symptoms may be difficult to distinguish from early signs of Huntington's disease, although the family history and course of Huntington's soon allow them to be differentiated. Finally, some mild symptoms, such as lip smacking and pill-rolling motions of the hands, may be seen in older individuals without other significant pathology.

Other late-onset movement disorders, specifically tardive dystonia and tardive akathisia, are less common but share many properties with TD, especially association with long-term exposure to antipsychotic medications. As the names indicate, they represent late-developing and persistent muscle cramps or restlessness similar to those seen more often early in treatment.

Although generally treated as a chronic condition, TD may follow a variety of courses. In general, symptoms show little progression after they occur and, in some cases, may spontaneously improve or remit altogether, despite continuation of antipsychotic treatment. Symptoms may be transiently suppressed by an increased dose of antipsychotic, which should

Tardive Dyskinesia **183**

not be mistaken for overall improvement because they will likely return within a brief time. Furthermore, symptoms may persist for months or years after the offending medication has been discontinued.

Recognition and Detection

TD's clinical presentation often includes disfiguring movements of the lips, tongue, or jaw; arrhythmic movements of the feet or hands; and postural movements of the neck and trunk. In contrast to the intentional writhing of akathisia, which is driven by subjective discomfort, TD occurs without voluntary awareness and can be consciously suppressed for brief periods, only to resume when attention is diverted elsewhere. Symptoms tend to worsen when patients are anxious or agitated.

TD is included in the "Medication-Induced Movement Disorders and Other Adverse Effects of Medication" chapter of DSM-5-TR, described as "abnormal, involuntary movements… that develop in association with the use of medications that block postsynaptic dopamine receptors" (American Psychiatric Association 2022, p. 814). Diagnostic criteria include a minimum of 3 months' exposure to the offending drug (1 month in older individuals), development of symptoms during or within 4 weeks of drug exposure, and persistence of symptoms for at least 4 weeks.

Culprit Medications

As noted earlier, both FGA and SGA medications are clearly associated with TD, with FGAs carrying the greater risk. Other dopaminergic drugs not usually classified as antipsychotics, including metoclopramide and prochlorperazine, have been implicated via the same mechanism. In contrast, little evidence indicates that anticholinergic drugs, such as benztropine and trihexyphenidyl, cause TD.

Much discussion and some useful data have been published regarding differences in risk among the various SGAs. Clozapine stands out in this group, can be acknowledged with confidence to carry low risk, and shows evidence of potential to treat TD caused by other antipsychotic medications. Conclusions about other SGAs are less certain. A common suggestion is that quetiapine, with its relatively low risk for other types of movement disorder, may carry lower risk of TD as well, but data supporting this view are sparse.

Assessment

DSM-5-TR includes no criteria regarding the level of abnormal movements, distress, or dysfunction required to make a diagnosis of TD. In the absence of more specific DSM-5 criteria, most expert consensus guidelines endorse the Abnormal Involuntary Movement Scale (AIMS) as the preferred instrument to assess and monitor the severity of TD symptoms in the clinical setting. Developed by the National Institute of Mental Health, the scale is validated, widely used, easy to administer, and available in the public domain (Maryland Department of Health 1976). It includes observer ratings of severity for seven body areas (muscles of facial expression, lips and perioral area, jaw, tongue, upper extremities, lower extremities, trunk) on a 5-point scale from 0 (none) to 4 (severe). Three items then use the same scale to assess global movement, incapacitation, and the patient's subjective distress. Two final items ask about dental issues as a possible confounding factor in assessment of the oral movements. The test takes only a few minutes and can be completed during a routine clinical visit. Despite the absence of specific anchors for the severity scores, clinicians' judgments show good interrater and test-retest reliability.

The motor components of the AIMS are assessed with the patient seated upright in a rigid chair and facing the examiner with their feet flat on the floor and hands resting on thighs or knees. The patient should remove any gum or candy from their mouth. The clinician should ask about any current problems with teeth or dentures. Abnormal movements may not occur immediately after a change in position; sufficient time must be allowed after each instruction for spontaneous movements to emerge. Abnormal movements may be suppressed by conscious effort if the patient is aware of what is being examined; clinicians should not call attention to exactly what they are looking for.

The clinician should

- Observe the patient sitting quietly, noting both global movement and each of the seven body regions.

- Ask the patient to sit with arms hanging down either between legs or over knees, again making both global and area-specific observations.
- Ask the patient to open their mouth to observe the tongue at rest, and then repeat the instruction.
- Ask the patient to protrude the tongue as the clinician looks for abnormalities in the movement; this step should be repeated.
- Ask the patient to tap the thumb to each finger of the right hand as fast as possible for 10–15 seconds and then do the same with the left hand to distract attention from other movements as facial and leg movements are observed.
- Flex and extend the patient's right arm and then the left.
- Observe the patient standing in profile with arms at sides.
- Ask the patient to face them with arms extended and palms down while observing the face, trunk, and legs.
- Have the patient walk a few steps and back as gait and hands are observed; this step should be repeated.

The global components are determined by overall observations combined with information from the patient and caregivers regarding impairment in function and degree of awareness and distress.

AIMS scores provide one critical element of the diagnosis. In the widely used Schooler-Kane criteria, a rating of at least 3 (moderate severity) in one body area or 2 (mild severity) in more than one area is sufficient for the diagnosis in a patient with at least 3 months of exposure to antipsychotic medications in whom no other basis for the movements can be identified (Schooler and Kane 1982). More recent guidelines expand this to suggest that even a rating of 2 in a single body area justifies consideration of "possible TD" (Caroff et al. 2020).

In clinical practice, screening all patients taking an antipsychotic at every clinical encounter should be considered the standard of care. On most occasions, this will be limited to observation during the interview for any atypical movements and questions about whether the patient or caregivers have noted such movements. Both positive and negative responses, including the location and intensity of any movements, should be recorded in the clinical note. A structured assessment involving the AIMS should be included if movements suggestive of TD are observed. Neurological consultation may be appropriate if symptoms appear atypical, there is a family history of movement disorders, or other neurological abnormalities are present. A series of positive AIMS tests over "at least a few weeks" confirms the diagnosis.

Management

The first factor to consider before discussion of treatment is the degree of distress and disability caused by the TD symptoms. Many mild cases do not cause significant concern to the patient and need only be monitored for progression. In all cases, the burden of TD must be weighed against the risks associated with available treatments. A frank discussion of these issues with the patient and family should precede any recommendations.

If treatment appears to be appropriate, it should begin with an assessment of the need for continued antipsychotics. For patients in whom the medication was initiated to address a transient or episodic disorder, such as bipolar mania, psychotic depression, or delirium, discontinuation of the offending agent should be considered. For disorders such as schizophrenia, for which continuity of antipsychotic treatment may be critical, careful consideration of a reduction in dose or transition to an agent with less potential for TD would be appropriate, particularly if an FGA is involved.

Clozapine has long been acknowledged to be an effective treatment for moderate to severe TD and may be a good option for any patient with an established need for antipsychotic medication to maintain stability whose TD would justify the additional side-effect burden of the drug. This approach has the advantage of potentially improving the antipsychotic response the patient experiences while reducing abnormal movements. In all cases, however, the benefits must be weighed against the inconvenience of frequent blood tests and increased risks of metabolic dysregulation, anticholinergic effects, cardiac complications, and severe neutropenia that accompany clozapine treatment.

Two vesicular monoamine transporter type 2 (VMAT2) inhibitors, deutetrabenazine and valbenazine, have been approved by the FDA for the treatment of TD. These agents block the uptake of dopamine into presynaptic vesicles, thereby reducing the overall level of dopamine available to postsynaptic receptors. This approach has long been used in the treatment of Huntington's disease with tetrabenazine, another medication of the same class.

Deutetrabenazine has shown moderate effects in patients who developed TD during antipsychotic treatment for either schizophrenia or a mood disorder (Teva 2022). In its clinical trials, patients typically showed about 35% reduction in TD symptoms, compared with 15% improvement with placebo, with about 35% of patients experiencing at least 50% improvement. Side effects in these studies were similar to those with placebo, but in similar studies involving patients with Huntington's disease, somnolence, diarrhea, fatigue, and insomnia all occurred at rates at least 5% higher than with placebo. Deutetrabenazine may be initiated at doses of 6 mg twice daily, titrated in weekly intervals at steps of 6 mg/day to a maximum of 48 mg/day. Doses should be taken with food, which increases absorption by 50%. The liver enzyme carbonyl reductase is required to convert the parent drug to its active metabolites, which reach peak concentrations 3–4 hours after dosing. The active compounds are cleared by hepatic cytochrome P450 2D6 (CYP2D6) with a half-life of 9–10 hours. The drug is contraindicated in patients with hepatic impairment.

Valbenazine has shown comparable results in its clinical trials, with about 30% reduction in AIMS scores, compared with no change for patients receiving placebo, and 40% of patients taking the active drug experiencing at least 50% reduction in their symptoms, compared with 10% of those in the control group (Neurocrine Biosciences 2021). Only somnolence was classified by the FDA as "common" when compared with placebo rates (10.9% vs. 4.2%), with parkinsonism occurring in 3% of patients compared with less than 1% in the placebo group. In a 48-week open-label study, improvement stabilized at 8 weeks and remained constant thereafter, but symptoms recurred in most patients after the drug was discontinued (Neurocrine Biosciences 2021). Valbenazine should be initiated at 40 mg daily and increased to 80 mg daily after 1 week. The higher dose showed superior performance in the clinical trials, but a dose of 40–60 mg daily may be appropriate in patients who develop side effects. The drug is absorbed in 30–60 minutes, with nearly 50% increase in absorption with a high-fat meal, although the manufacturer has no recommendation regarding this. An active metabolite has negligible effect on its overall function, and both are cleared by the liver, the parent compound via CYP3A4/5 and the metabolite by CYP2D6. Dose reduction is recommended for patients with hepatic impairment.

Although neither of these drugs fully controls TD symptoms, the number needed to treat for a 50% improvement with either of them is 3–4, an excellent rate for a disorder as difficult to address as TD has been historically. Combined with other interventions, they provide a significant improvement over previously available treatment.

Some evidence supports the use of a few other medications. Ginkgo biloba extract has shown modest benefit in a series of placebo-controlled studies, with good tolerability (Zheng et al. 2016). On the basis of one older study, amantadine may have moderate beneficial effects (Angus et al. 1997). Mixed evidence has been presented for clonazepam, which may be most effective in patients whose movements are triggered or worsened by anxiety (Bergman et al. 2018; Bhidayasiri et al. 2018).

A remarkable number and variety of other medications have been recommended for TD, including acetazolamide, α-methyldopa, baclofen, botulinum toxin type A, bromocriptine, buspirone, diltiazem, eicosapentaenoic acid, flupentixol, fluperlapine, galantamine, levetiracetam, melatonin, nifedipine, reserpine, selegiline, sulpiride, thiamine, thiopropazate, vitamin E, and vitamin B_6. None of these treatments have been consistently effective in controlled trials (Bhidayasiri et al. 2013).

Several small studies have reported success in treatment-refractory cases of TD with bilateral deep brain stimulation of the globus pallidus (Gruber et al. 2018), and a trial of repetitive transcranial magnetic stimulation of the motor cortex has likewise shown promise (Khedr et al. 2019). Although these studies consistently cite their results as being applicable to TD, most patients in these trials were diagnosed with a variety of tardive motor syndromes, not just TD, for which these invasive treatments have only occasionally been used.

Follow-Up Management

Patients remain at risk for TD beyond the acute phases of the disorder and its treatment, so most steps taken in the acute management of TD will need to be maintained, and possibly increased, thereafter. Changes in antipsychotic medication and dose should be continued unless recurrence of psychotic symptoms or resurgence of TD requires an adjustment. Studies of patients taking deutetrabenazine (Teva 2022) or valbenazine (Marder et al. 2019; Neurocrine Biosciences 2021) for up to 1 year reported high rates of relapse with discontinuation of these medications. These medications appear to be well tolerated throughout that period, and there is no clear contraindication to their long-term continuation. Although anticholinergic drugs do not appear to cause TD, they may worsen some symptoms, and some expert guidelines recommend their avoidance.

A pattern of routine observation and questions regarding TD at all clinical visits, accompanied by a full AIMS assessment at least quarterly, is appropriate to monitor for symptom progression. The overall severity of the disorder as assessed by the three AIMS global judgment scores provides a critical component of routine monitoring. It allows clear documentation of the onset and progression of the disorder, informs important treatment decisions, and provides assessment of treatment efficacy.

Conclusion

TD has long been an inevitable risk of maintenance antipsychotic treatment, with few effective options available to address troublesome symptoms. The introduction of SGAs has reduced but has not fully alleviated that risk. The recent development of effective medications to reduce TD symptoms has added important tools with which all clinicians should become familiar. Equally important is a realistic appraisal of the outcomes of those treatments and appropriate acknowledgment to patients and their caregivers of the risks associated with antipsychotic use.

Key Points

Tardive dyskinesia is a common and often serious side effect of long-term use of antipsychotic and other dopaminergic medications that should be assessed at all routine clinic visits.

Familiarity with and routine use of the Abnormal Involuntary Movement Scale (AIMS) will aid in the diagnosis and monitoring of tardive dyskinesia onset, progression, and response to treatment.

Treatment begins with consideration of possible changes in antipsychotic medication treatment, including discontinuation, dose reduction, and transition to an alternative drug, including clozapine.

Use of vesicular monoamine transporter type 2 (VMAT2) inhibitors is recommended when adjustment of the antipsychotic medication is inappropriate or ineffective.

References

American Psychiatric Association: Diagnostic and Statistical Manual of Mental Disorders, 5th Edition, Text Revision. Washington, DC, American Psychiatric Association, 2022

Angus S, Sugars J, Boltezar , et al: A controlled trial of amantadine hydrochloride and neuroleptics in the treatment of tardive dyskinesia. J Clin Psychopharmacol 17(2):88–91, 1997 10950469

Bergman H, Rathbone J, Agarwal V, Soares-Weiser K: Antipsychotic reduction and/or cessation and antipsychotics as specific treatments for tardive dyskinesia. Cochrane Database Syst Rev 2(2):CD000459, 2018 29409162

Bhidayasiri R, Fahn S, Weiner WJ, et al: Evidence-based guideline: treatment of tardive syndromes: report of the Guideline Development Subcommittee of the American Academy of Neurology. Neurology 81(5):463–469, 2013 23897874

Bhidayasiri R, Jitkritsadakul O, Friedman JH, Fahn S: Updating the recommendations for treatment of tardive syndromes: a systematic review of new evidence and practical treatment algorithm. J Neurol Sci 389:67–75, 2018 29454493

Carbon M, Hsieh C-H, Kane JM, Correll CU: Tardive dyskinesia prevalence in the period of second-generation antipsychotic use: a meta-analysis. J Clin Psychiatry 78:e264–e278, 2017 28146614

Carbon M, Kane JM, Leucht S, Correll CU: Tardive dyskinesia risk with first- and second-generation antipsychotics in comparative randomized controlled trials: a meta-analysis. World Psychiatry 17(3):330–340, 2018 30192088

Caroff SN, Citrome L, Meyer J, et al: A modified Delphi consensus study of the screening, diagnosis, and treatment of tardive dyskinesia. J Clin Psychiatry 81(2):50–60, 2020 31995677

Gruber D, Südmeyer M, Deuschl G, et al: Neurostimulation in tardive dystonia/dyskinesia: a delayed start, sham stimulation-controlled randomized trial. Brain Stimul 11(6):1368–1377, 2018 30249417

Jeste DV, Caligiuri MP, Paulsen JS, et al: Risk of tardive dyskinesia in older patients: a prospective longitudinal study of 266 outpatients. Arch Gen Psychiatry 52(9):756–765, 1995 7654127

Khedr EM, Al Fawal B, Abdelwarith A, et al: Repetitive transcranial magnetic stimulation for treatment of tardive syndromes: double randomized clinical trial. J Neural Transm (Vienna) 126(2):183–191, 2019 30317532

Marder SR, Singer C, Lindenmayer JP, et al: A phase 3, 1-year, open-label trial of valbenazine in adults with tardive dyskinesia. J Clin Psychopharmacol 39(6):620–627, 2019 31688452

Maryland Department of Health: Abnormal Involuntary Movement Scale. 1976. Available at: https://health.maryland.gov/mmcp/pap/docs/Antipsychotic%20Review%20Programs/Abnormal%20Involuntary%20Movement%20Scale.pdf#search=Abnormal%20Involuntary%20Movement%20Scal. Accessed November 2, 2022.

Neurocrine Biosciences: Ingrezza package insert. 2021. Available at: www.neurocrine.com/assets/INGREZZA-full-Prescribing-Information.pdf#page=18. Accessed November 3, 2022.

Schooler NR, Kane JM: Research diagnoses for tardive dyskinesia. Arch Gen Psychiatry 39(4):486–487, 1982 6121550

Tarsy D, Baldessarini RJ: Epidemiology of tardive dyskinesia: is risk declining with modern antipsychotics? Mov Disord 21(5):589–598, 2006 16532448

Teva: Austedo package insert. 2022. Available at: https://www.austedo.com/globalassets/austedo/prescribing-information.pdf. Accessed November 3, 2022.

Woerner MG, Correll CU, Alvir JMJ, et al: Incidence of tardive dyskinesia with risperidone or olanzapine in the elderly: results from a 2-year, prospective study in antipsychotic-naïve patients. Neuropsychopharmacology 36(8):1738–1746, 2011 21508932

Zheng W, Xiang YQ, Ng CH, et al: Extract of Ginkgo biloba for tardive dyskinesia: meta-analysis of randomized controlled trials. Pharmacopsychiatry 49(3):107–111, 2016 26979525

Index

Abnormal Involuntary Movement Scale (AIMS), 53, 185–187, 190

Absolute neutrophil count (ANC), 21. *See also* Agranulocytosis, with clozapine and other psychotropic medications

Acetaminophen + hydrocodone, combined with opioids, 31

Acetazolamide, TD and, 189

Acetylsalicylic acid + oxycodone, combined with opioids, 31

Acid. *See* Lysergic acid diethylamide

Acute dystonia
  assessment of, 4–6
  culprit medications and, 3–4
  follow-up management of, 7
  induced by psychotropics, 8
  management of, 6–7
  manifestation of, 2, 8
  mechanism of action of, 1, 8
  medication-induced, 3
  overview, 1–3
  reactions to, 1
  recognition and detection of, 3
  risk factors for, 2–3, 8
  second-line therapy for, 6–7
  sudden death and, 4
  symptoms of, 4–6
  treatment of, 6–7, 8

Addiction
  culprit substances and medications
    cannabinoids, 172–173
    ethanol, 168–170
    nicotine and cigarette smoking, 173–175
    psychedelics, 175–176
    stimulants, 170–172
  follow-up management of, 176
  overview, 167

ADEs (adverse drug events), 125. *See also* Polypharmacy, acute side effects of

ADH (antidiuretic hormone), 81. *See also* Hyponatremia

β-Adrenergic-blocking agents, stimulants and, 171

Adverse drug events (ADEs), 125. *See also* Polypharmacy, acute side effects of

Age. *See* Elderly

Agitated Behavior Scale, 16

Agitation
  assessment of, 15–16
  culprit medications and, 11–15
    antidepressants, 11–12
    antipsychotics, 12–13
    benzodiazepines, 14
    mood stabilizers, 13–14
    nonbenzodiazepine receptor agonists, 14
  description of, 11

Agitation *(continued)*
    follow-up management of, 17
    management of, 16–17
    overview, 11
    recognition and detection of, 11
Agomelatine, discontinuation of, 55
Agranulocytosis, with clozapine and other psychotropic medications
    assessment of, 24–25
        clinical setting for, 24
        complete blood count, 24–25, 26
        initial evaluation of, 24
    culprit medications, 22–24
        anticonvulsants, 23
        antidepressants, 23
        mood stabilizers, 23
    definition of, 21
    etiology and pathogenesis of, 23–24
    fatality rate of, 21, 22, 25
    follow-up management of, 25–26
    incidence of, 21–22
    infection and, 25
    management of, 25
    overview, 21–22
    presentation of, 24
    psychoeducation about, 26
    recognition and detection of, 22
    risk factors for, 26
    stabilization of, 25
AIMS (Abnormal Involuntary Movement Scale), 53, 185
Akathisia, antipsychotic-induced, 16
Alanine transaminase (ALT), 64
Alcohol, addiction to, 168

Alcohol use disorder, 14
    disulfiram for treatment of, 169
Alprazolam
    combined with opioids, 31
    risk of seizures with, 151
ALT (alanine transaminase), 64
Amantadine, NMS and, 93
American Geriatrics Society Beers Criteria for Potentially Inappropriate Medication Use in Older Adults, 82, 83, 126, 129, 131. *See also* Polypharmacy, acute side effects of
Amitriptyline
    Brugada syndrome and, 41
    ethanol and, 168
    hepatotoxicity and, 64
    nicotine and, 173
Amoxapine, agranulocytosis and, 23
Amphetamines
    addiction to, 170
    coronary vasospasm and, 48
    during pregnancy, 139
    serotonin syndrome and, 159
ANC (absolute neutrophil count), 21. *See also* Agranulocytosis, with clozapine and other psychotropic medications
Angiotensin converting enzyme inhibitors
    for management of myocarditis, 46
    for management of noninflammatory cardiomyopathy, 47

Antibiotics, serotonin
syndrome and, 159
Anticholinergic Cognitive
Burden Scale, 127
Anticholinergics
anticholinergic burden,
127
muscarinic receptors, 126
NMS and, 93
polypharmacy, acute side
effects of, 126–127
Anticonvulsant medications
agranulocytosis and, 23
discontinuation of, 54–55
assessment of, 54
management of, 54–55
recognition and
detection of, 54
Antidepressants
agitation and, 11–12
agranulocytosis and, 23
as cause of SIADH or
hyponatremia,
83–84, 88
discontinuation of, 55–57
assessment of, 56
brain zaps and, 55
follow-up management
of, 57
management of, 56–57
persistent
postwithdrawal
disorder, 56
rebound symptoms, 56
withdrawal symptoms,
55–56
hepatotoxicity and,
64–65
intentional overdose of,
117
overdose of, 122
during pregnancy, 140
risk of seizures with, 149
Antidiuretic hormone
(ADH), 81. *See also*
Hyponatremia

Antiemetics
acute dystonia and, 4
NMS and, 93
Antiepileptic drugs
anticholinergic effects and,
126–127
as cause of SIADH or
hyponatremia,
84–85, 88
during pregnancy, 142
Antihistamines,
anticholinergic effects
and, 126–127
Antihypertensive agents, for
management of
serotonin syndrome, 163
Antimuscarinic drugs, for
management of
antipsychotic overdose,
120
Antiparkinsonian drugs
anticholinergic effects and,
126–127
withdrawal and NMS, 93
Antipsychotic medications
agitation and, 12–13
anticholinergic effects and,
126–127
as cause of SIADH or
hyponatremia, 83, 85,
88
delirium and, 13
discontinuation of, 52–53
assessment of, 53
follow-up management
of, 53
management of, 53
recognition and
detection of, 52
persistent postwith-
drawal disor-
der, 52
rebound symptoms, 52
withdrawal
symptoms, 52
ethanol and, 169

Antipsychotic medications
(continued)
extrapyramidal side effects
of, 119
nicotine and, 173–174
polypharmacy, acute side
effects of, 128–129
during pregnancy, 139
risk of seizures with,
150–151
TD and, 187
Antivirals, serotonin
syndrome and, 159
Anxiety
associated with
bupropion, 12
opioids and, 35
in women, 135
Anxiolytics, risk of seizures
with, 151
Apgar scores, 143
Aripiprazole
acute dystonia and, 4
oculogyric crisis and, 105
toxicity from, 121
Asymptomatic alanine
transaminase (ALT),
64
Atomoxetine, during
pregnancy, 139
Atrioventricular (AV) block
assessment of, 44
culprit medications, 44
description of, 43
follow-up management of,
45
management of, 44
recognition and detection
of, 43–44
types of, 43
Atypical antidepressants,
agitation and, 12
AV. See Atrioventricular
block
Avanafil, visual disturbances
related to, 107–108

Baclofen
NMS and, 93
TD and, 189
Barbiturates, ethanol and,
169
Barnes Akathisia Rating
Scale, 16
Benzodiazepines, 116–117
agitation and, 14
as allosteric modulators,
127
AV block and, 44
in combination with
opioids
assessment of, 31–32
culprit medications, 31
follow-up management
of, 35
incidence, 29–30
management of, 32–35
overview, 29–30
recognition and
detection of
toxicity, 30–31
discontinuation of, 57–59,
162–163
assessment of, 58
follow-up management
of, 59
management of, 58–59
overview, 57
recognition and
detection of,
57–58
persistent postwith-
drawal disor-
der, 58
rebound symptoms,
58
withdrawal
symptoms,
57–58
dosage, 36
ethanol and, 169
false-negative tests for,
33–34

flexible tapers for, 34
hepatotoxicity and, 68
for management of acute
    dystonia, 6–7
methadone and, 31
NMS and, 95
ocular side effects of, 103
polypharmacy, acute side
    effects of, 127–128
during pregnancy, 139–140
risk factors and, 34, 36
risk of seizures with, 151
stable, low-dose therapy,
    31
for treatment of serotonin
    toxicity, 123
Benztropine
    for follow-up management
        of acute dystonia, 7
    for management of acute
        dystonia, 6
    for management of
        antipsychotic
        overdose, 120
    for management of
        oculogyric crisis, 105
Bipolar depression
    pramipexole for treatment
        of, 14
    relapse of, 55
β-Blockers
    AV block and, 44
    for management of
        myocarditis, 46
    for management of
        noninflammatory
        cardiomyopathy, 47
Blue tinge, 107
Botulinum toxin type A, TD
    and, 189
Bradykinesia, 119
Brain zaps, 55
Bromocriptine
    for management of
        antipsychotic
        overdose, 120

NMS and, 95
TD and, 189
Brugada syndrome
    assessment of, 42
    culprit medications, 41
    description of, 41
    follow-up management of,
        42
    management of, 42
    recognition and detection
        of, 41
Buccolingual crisis, 4
Bupropion
    addiction to, 170
    associated with anxiety,
        12
    AV block and, 44
    as cause of SIADH or
        hyponatremia, 84, 87
    discontinuation of, 55
    ethanol and, 168
    hepatotoxicity and, 64, 65
    nicotine and, 173
    overdose of, 116
    during pregnancy, 137
    risk of seizures with, 149,
        152
Bush-Francis Catatonia
    Rating Scale, 16
Buspirone
    risk of seizures with,
        151
    serotonin syndrome and,
        159
    TD and, 189
Butyrophenones, oculogyric
    crisis and, 105

Caffeine, risk of seizures
    with, 152
Calcium channel blockers
    AV block and, 44
    for management of
        coronary vasospasm,
        48
Cannabidiol (CBD), 172

Cannabinoids, addiction to, 177
  assessment of, 173
  management of, 173
  recognition and detection of, 172
Cannabis
  Brugada syndrome and, 41
  coronary vasospasm and, 48
Carbamazepine
  agitation and, 12–13
  agranulocytosis and, 23
  AV block and, 44
  Brugada syndrome and, 41
  as cause of SIADH or hyponatremia, 83, 84–85, 88
  discontinuation of, 54
  ocular side effects of, 103
  oculogyric crisis and, 105
  pigmentary retinal deposits and, 107
  during pregnancy, 138
  ventricular conduction delay and, 45
Cardiac emergencies
  atrioventricular block, 43–45
  Brugada syndrome, 41–42
  coronary vasospasm, 47–48
  myocarditis, 46–47
  noninflammatory cardiomyopathy, 47
  overview, 39
  psychiatry and cardiology collaboration for, 49
  serotonin syndrome and, 161–162
  sick sinus syndrome, 42–43
  torsades de pointes, 39–41
  ventricular conduction delay, 45
Carvedilol, AV block and, 44
Cataracts. See Pigmentary cataract deposits

Catatonia, 5–6, 92
CBC. See Complete blood count
CBD (cannabidiol), 172
CBT, for management of chronic pain and chronic anxiety, 35
CDC. See Centers for Disease Control and Prevention
Centers for Disease Control and Prevention (CDC), 31
  recommendation guidelines for management of benzodiazepines and opioids, 32–35
Chlordiazepoxide
  combined with opioids, 31
  pigmentary retinal deposits and, 107
Chlorpromazine
  acute dystonia and, 3
  hepatotoxicity and, 66
  ocular side effects of, 100
  pigmentary cataract deposits and, 106
  polypharmacy, acute side effects of, 129
  risk of seizures with, 150
  TdP and, 40
Choreiform movements, 92
Ciprofloxacin, serotonin syndrome and, 159
Citalopram
  association with D_2 receptor–blocking agents, 1
  AV block and, 44
  hepatotoxicity and, 64
  NMS and, 93
  ocular side effects of, 101
  during pregnancy, 136
  TdP and, 40
Clevidipine, dosing, 78

Clomipramine
  agranulocytosis and, 23
  Brugada syndrome and,
    41
Clonazepam
  combined with opioids, 31
  for management of acute
    dystonia, 7
  risk of seizures with, 151
  TD and, 189
Clozapine. *See also*
    Agranulocytosis, with
    clozapine and other
    psychotropic
    medications
  AV block and, 44
  hepatotoxicity and, 66
  management of toxicity
    from, 174–175
  myocarditis and, 46
  nicotine and, 174
  NMS and, 92
  noninflammatory
    cardiomyopathy and,
    47
  polypharmacy, acute side
    effects of, 129
  risk of seizures with,
    150–151, 152
  TD and, 187
Cocaine
  addiction to, 170
  Brugada syndrome and,
    41
  coronary vasospasm and,
    48
  hypertensive crisis and, 77
  serotonin syndrome and,
    159
  ventricular conduction
    delay and, 45
Codeine, combined with
    opioids, 31
Cohen-Mansfield Agitation
    Inventory Observational
    Tool, 16

Complete blood count (CBC),
    for assessment of
    agranulocytosis, 24–25, 26
Coronary vasospasm
  assessment of, 48
  culprit medications, 48
  description of, 47
  follow-up management of,
    48
  management of, 48
  recognition and detection
    of, 48
Corticosteroids
  for management of
    myocarditis, 46
  for management of
    noninflammatory
    cardiomyopathy, 47
Counseling, about risks of in
    utero medication
    exposure, 141
Cycloplegia, 101
  assessment of, 104
  culprit medications, 104
  description of, 103–104
  follow-up management of,
    104
  management of, 104
  recognition and detection
    of, 104
CYP. *See* Cytochrome P450
CYP2D6 inhibitors
  AV block and, 44
  psychedelics and, 175
  serotonin syndrome and,
    159
CYP enzymes, nicotine and,
    173–174
Cyproheptadine, for
    management of
    serotonin syndrome,
    163, 172
Cytochrome isoform 2D6, 65
Cytochrome P450 (CYP),
    158–159
  cannabis and, 172

D_2/D_3 agonist, 14
Dantrolene
    for management of
        antipsychotic
        overdose, 120
    NMS and, 95
Death. *See also* Toxicity
    from benzodiazepines in
        combination with
        opioids, 29–30
    Brugada syndrome and, 41
    from stimulants, 171
    sudden, 4
Deep brain stimulation, TD
    and, 189
Delirium, antipsychotic
    medications and, 13
Delirium Rating Scale, 16
Dementia, polypharmacy,
    acute side effects of, 129
Depression
    treatment for, 88–89
    in women, 135
Desipramine
    Brugada syndrome and,
        41
Desmopressin, as cause of
    SIADH or
    hyponatremia, 83
Desvenlafaxine
    hepatotoxicity and, 64, 65
    during pregnancy, 136
Deutetrabenazine
    for management of
        antipsychotic
        medications, 53
    TD and, 187, 188
Dexmethylphenidate,
    coronary vasospasm
    and, 48
Dextroamphetamine
    coronary vasospasm and,
        48
Dextromethorphan,
    serotonin syndrome
    and, 159

Diazepam
    combined with opioids, 31
    hepatotoxicity and, 68
    for management of acute
        dystonia, 6–7
    for management of
        serotonin syndrome,
        163
    risk of seizures with, 151
Dietary supplements,
    serotonin syndrome
    and, 159
Diltiazem, TD and, 189
Diphenhydramine
    for management of acute
        dystonia, 6
    for management of
        antipsychotic
        overdose, 120
    for management of
        oculogyric crisis, 105
Disulfiram, ethanol and, 169
Diuretics
    as cause of SIADH or
        hyponatremia, 83
    for management of
        myocarditis, 46
    for management of
        noninflammatory
        cardiomyopathy, 47
Domperidone, NMS and, 93
Donepezil, hepatotoxicity
    and, 68
Dopamine D_2 receptor–
    blocking agents
    as cause of SIADH or
        hyponatremia, 85
    for treatment of AV block,
        44
Dose dumping, 169
Dosulepin, NMS and, 93
DSM-5-TR
    description of TD, 184
    diagnosis of TD, 185
Duloxetine
    ethanol and, 168

hepatotoxicity and, 64
nicotine and, 173
during pregnancy, 137
Dysarthria, 4
Dysautonomia, 92
Dystonia, 1, 104. *See also*
  Acute dystonia;
  Oculogyric crisis
  differential diagnosis of, 5
  incidence of, 2
  location of, 8
  management of, 120
  risk factors for, 8
  symptoms of, 2

Ecstasy. *See* 3,4-Methylenedi-
  oxymethamphetamine
ECT (electroconvulsive
  therapy), for NMS, 95
Edinburgh Postnatal
  Depression Scale, 140
Education, about risks of in
  utero medication
  exposure, 141
EEG (electroencephalogram),
  153
Eicosapentaenoic acid, TD
  and, 189
Elderly. *See also*
  Hyponatremia;
  Polypharmacy, acute
  side effects of
  comorbidities in, 129–130
  incidence of dystonia in, 2
  risk of agranulocytosis in,
  6
Electroconvulsive therapy
  (ECT), for NMS, 95
Electroencephalogram (EEG),
  153
End-organ damage, 79
End-stage renal disease
  (ESRD), serotonin
  syndrome and,
  159, 160
Ephedra, addiction to, 170

Ephedrine, hypertensive
  crisis and, 77
Epilepsy, 85
Epinephrine
  for treatment of AV block, 44
  for treatment of TdP, 41
EPS (extrapyramidal side
  effects), 119
Erectile dysfunction, 107
Ergotamine, serotonin
  syndrome and, 159
Escitalopram
  ethanol and, 168
  hepatotoxicity and, 64
  ocular side effects of, 101
  oculogyric crisis and, 105
  during pregnancy, 136
  TdP and, 40
Esmolol, for management of
  serotonin syndrome, 163
ESRD (end-stage renal
  disease), serotonin
  syndrome and, 159, 160
Ethanol
  addiction to, 177
  assessment of, 169
  management of,
  169–170
  recognition and
  detection of,
  168–169
Ethosuximide,
  agranulocytosis and, 23
Extrapyramidal side effects
  (EPS), 119
Eyes. *See also* Pigmentary
  cataract deposits;
  Pigmentary retinal
  deposits; Psychotropic
  medications, ocular side
  effects of
  abnormal pigmentation of,
  100
  dilation of pupils, 101
  double vision of, 102–103
  farsighted vision, 101

Fentanyl
combined with opioids, 31
serotonin syndrome and,
159
FGAs. *See* First-generation
agents; First-generation
antipsychotics
First-generation agents
(FGAs)
agitation and, 12–13
hepatotoxicity and, 66
polypharmacy, acute side
effects of, 128–129
First-generation
antipsychotics (FGAs),
52
TD and, 181–182
Fluoxetine
AV block and, 4
as cause of SIADH or
hyponatremia, 84
discontinuation of, 56–57
ocular side effects of, 101
during pregnancy, 136
serotonin syndrome and,
159
Flupentixol, TD and, 189
Fluperlapine, TD and, 189
Fluphenazine
acute dystonia and, 3, 4
agranulocytosis and, 23
hepatotoxicity and, 66
Flurazepam, combined with
opioids, 31
Fluvoxamine
hepatotoxicity and, 64
nicotine and, 173
ocular side effects of, 101
during pregnancy, 136
Folic acid, during pregnancy,
142
Food, hypertensive crisis
and, 77

Gabapentin, hepatotoxicity
and, 68

Galantamine
hepatotoxicity and, 68
TD and, 189
G-CSF. *See* Granulocyte
colony-stimulating
factor
Generalized tonic-clonic
seizures (GTCS), 147,
148
Ginkgo biloba, TD and, 189
Glaucoma
acute angle-closure,
100–102
description of, 100–101
medication-associated, 101
recognition and detection
of, 101
testing, 102
Granulocyte colony-
stimulating factor
(G-CSF)
agranulocytosis and, 23–24
lithium and, 23
GTCS (generalized tonic-
clonic seizures), 147, 148
"Guideline for Prescribing
Opioids for Chronic
Pain," 31

Haloperidol
acute dystonia and, 3, 4
agranulocytosis and, 22–23
nicotine and, 174
TdP and, 40
Heidelberg Retina
Tomograph, 100
Hematopoietic growth
factors, in management
of agranulocytosis, 25
Hepatotoxicity
antidepressants and, 64–65
antipsychotics and, 66–67
benzodiazepines and, 68
definition of, 71
mood stabilizers and,
67–68

nonbenzodiazepine
receptor agonists
and, 68
Hunter Serotonin Toxicity
Criteria, 158, 165, 171
Huntington's disease, 183,
187
Hydrocodone, combined
with opioids, 31
Hydromorphone, combined
with opioids, 31
Hyperammonemia, agitation
and, 14
Hyperbolic tapering,
anticonvulsants and, 57
Hypercalcemia, lithium and,
14
Hyperpyrexia, 92
NMS and, 95
Hypersensitivity syndrome,
67
Hypertensive crisis,
associated with MAOIs
assessment of, 77–78
culprit medications, 77
definition of, 76, 79
follow-up management of,
78
foods and, 77
illegal drugs and, 77
management of, 78
overview, 75–76
recognition and detection
of, 76–77
Hypocalcemia, 5
Hyponatremia, 12
adverse outcomes of, 82
assessment of, 86
culprit medications and
other causes, 83–86
antidepressants, 83–84
antiepileptic drugs,
84–85
antipsychotics, 85
psychogenic polydipsia,
85–86

definition of, 81
discontinuation syndrome
and, 86–87
follow-up management of,
87–88
management of, 86–87
onset of, 84
overview, 81–82
recognition and detection
of, 82–83
risk factors for, 88
Hypothyroidism, lithium
and, 14

Iloperidone, TdP and, 40
Imipramine
agranulocytosis and, 23
hepatotoxicity and, 64
nicotine and, 173
Indole, overdose of, 121
Infants
exposure to psychotropic
medications, 144
PPHN and, 136
Infection, due to
granulocytosis, 25
Intravenous Mg^{2+}, TdP and,
40
Irritability. *See also* Agitation
description of, 11
Isocarboxazid, hypertensive
crisis and, 75

Ketamine, risk of seizures
with, 150
Khat, addiction to, 170
Kidneys, 81. *See also*
Hyponatremia
serotonin syndrome and,
161

Lamotrigine
agitation and, 13–14
Brugada syndrome and, 41
discontinuation of, 54

Lamotrigine *(continued)*
  management during
    pregnancy, 142
  myocarditis and, 46
  ocular side effects of, 103
  during pregnancy, 138
  ventricular conduction
    delay and, 45
Laryngeal dystonia, 7, 8
Laryngospasm, 4
Lennox-Gastaut syndrome,
  148. *See also* Seizures
Leukocytosis, serotonin
  syndrome and, 161
Levetiracetam
  hepatotoxicity and, 67
  TD and, 189
Levodopa, NMS and, 93
Levomilnacipran, during
  pregnancy, 137
LFTs (liver function tests),
  63, 71
Lisdexamfetamine, coronary
  vasospasm and, 48
Lithium
  agitation and, 13–14
  AV block and, 44
  Brugada syndrome and, 41
  contraindication with
    NMS, 96
  discontinuation of, 53–54,
    143
    assessment of, 54
    follow-up management
      of, 54
    management of, 54
    recognition and
      detection of,
      53–54
  exposure to newborns,
    143
  granulocyte colony-
    stimulating factor
    and, 23
  hepatotoxicity and, 68
  hypercalcemia and, 14

hypothyroidism and, 14
management during
  pregnancy, 142–143
noninflammatory
  cardiomyopathy and,
  47
ocular side effects of, 103
overdose of, 111
during pregnancy,
  137–138, 142, 144
risk of seizures with, 150
sick sinus syndrome and,
  43
toxicity, 14, 15, 117, 122
Liver, 63–64. *See also*
  Hepatotoxicity
  assessment of, 69
  cytochrome P450 system,
    128
  ethanol and, 168
  fatal damage to, 68
  hepatic failure, 70
  injury to, 65, 67, 68
Liver function tests (LFTs),
  63, 71
Long-acting nitroglycerin, for
  management of
  coronary vasospasm, 48
Lorazepam
  combined with opioids, 31
  for management of acute
    dystonia, 6–7
  for management of
    oculogyric crisis, 105
  NMS and, 95
  risk of seizures with, 151
Loxapine
  agranulocytosis and, 23
  Brugada syndrome and, 41
LSD (lysergic acid
  diethylamide), addiction
  to, 175
Lurasidone, overdose of, 121
Lysergic acid diethylamide
  (LSD; acid), addiction to,
  175

Magic mushrooms.
    See Psilocybin
Major depressive disorder,
    pramipexole for
    treatment of, 14
MAOIs. *See* Monoamine
    oxidase inhibitors
MDMA. *See* 3,4-Methylenedi-
    oxymethamphetamine
Melatonin, TD and, 189
Memantine, hepatotoxicity
    and, 68
Mental status, altered, 92
Meperidine, serotonin
    syndrome and, 159
Mephenytoin,
    agranulocytosis and, 23
Mesoridazine, TdP and, 40
Methadone
    benzodiazepines and, 31
    combined with opioids, 31
    hepatotoxicity and, 68
    serotonin syndrome and,
        159
    TdP and, 40
Methamphetamine, coronary
    vasospasm and, 48
α-Methyldopa, TD and, 189
3,4-Methylenedioxymetham-
    phetamine (MDMA)
    psychedelics and, 175, 177
    serotonin syndrome and,
        159
Methylphenidate
    coronary vasospasm and,
        48
    ethanol and, 169
    during pregnancy, 139
    risk of seizures with, 151
    stimulants and, 171
Metoclopramide
    acute dystonia and, 4
    TD and, 184
Metoprolol, AV block and, 44
Mianserin, discontinuation
    of, 55

Mirtazapine
    agranulocytosis and, 23
    as cause of SIADH or
        hyponatremia, 83
    discontinuation of, 55
    hepatotoxicity and, 65
    overdose of, 116
    during pregnancy, 137
    serotonin syndrome and,
        159
Mobitz type I (Wenckebach)
    AV block, 43, 44
    treatment of, 44
Mobitz type II AV block, 43,
    44
    treatment of, 44
Monoamine oxidase
    inhibitors (MAOIs)
    agitation and, 12
    agranulocytosis and, 23
    associated with
        hypertensive crisis,
        75–79
    dosing, 78
    ethanol and, 168
    mechanism of action of,
        75
    NMS and, 93
    nutrition and, 78
    risk of seizures with,
        149–150, 152
    serotonin syndrome and,
        159
    stimulants and, 170
Mood stabilizers
    agitation and, 13–14
    agranulocytosis and, 23
    discontinuation of, 53–55
    hepatotoxicity and, 67–68
    risk of seizures with, 150
    stimulants and, 170–171
Morphine, combined with
    opioids, 31
Morphine sulfate, for
    management of
    coronary vasospasm, 48

Movement disorders.
    See Tardive dyskinesia
Muscarinic receptors, 126
Muscle relaxants, for
    management of
    serotonin syndrome, 164
Mydriasis, 101
    assessment of, 104
    culprit medications, 104
    description of, 103–104
    follow-up management of,
        104
    management of, 104
    recognition and detection
        of, 104
Myocarditis
    assessment of, 46
    culprit medications, 46
    description of, 46
    endomyocardial biopsy for
        diagnosis of, 46
    follow-up management of,
        46–47
    management of, 46
    recognition and detection
        of, 46

Naloxone (Narcan), 34
Naltrexone, hepatotoxicity
    and, 68
Narcan (naloxone), 34
Narcotic analgesics,
    polypharmacy, acute
    side effects of, 128
Nebivolol, AV block and, 44
Nefazodone, hepatotoxicity
    and, 64, 65
Neuroleptic malignant
    syndrome (NMS)
    agitation and, 13
    assessment of, 15, 93–94
    culprit medications, 92–93
    diagnosis of, 93–94, 96
    EPS and, 119
    follow-up management of,
        96

incidence, 91, 92
    as life-threatening
        emergency, 96
    management of, 94–95, 97
    mechanism of action of, 91
    mortality of, 92
    overview, 91–92
    prognosis, 96
    recognition and detection
        of, 92
    restarting antipsychotic
        treatment after
        resolution of, 97
    risk factors for, 91–92
Neutropenia. *See also*
        Agranulocytosis, with
        clozapine and other
        psychotropic
        medications
    definition of, 21
Nicotine and cigarette
    smoking
    addiction to, 177
    assessment of, 174
    management of,
        174–175
    recognition and
        detection of,
        173–174
    electronic delivery of, 174
Nifedipine, TD and, 189
Nitroglycerine, for
    management of
    coronary vasospasm, 48
Nitroprusside, for
    management of
    serotonin syndrome, 163
NMS. *See* Neuroleptic
    malignant syndrome
Nonbenzodiazepine receptor
    agonists
    agitation and, 14
    hepatotoxicity and, 68
Nonbenzodiazepine
    sedative-hypnotics,
    ethanol and, 169

Noninflammatory
    cardiomyopathy
    assessment of, 47
    culprit medications, 47
    description of, 47
    follow-up management of,
        47
    management of, 47
    recognition and detection
        of, 47
Nonprescription drugs
    addiction to, 176
    stimulants and, 171
Nortriptyline
    agranulocytosis and, 23
    Brugada syndrome and, 41
Nutrition, MAOIs and, 78
Nystagmus, ocular side
    effects of, 103

Oculogyric crisis, 6–7.
    See also Dystonia
    assessment of, 105
    culprit medications, 105
    description of, 104–105
    follow-up management of,
        105
    management of, 105
    recognition and detection
        of, 105
Olanzapine
    acute dystonia and, 4
    hepatotoxicity and, 66
    myocarditis and, 46
    nicotine and, 174
    oculogyric crisis and, 105
    risk of seizures with, 150
Opioids
    anxiety and, 35
    in combination with
        benzodiazepines
        assessment of, 31–32
        culprit medications, 31
        follow-up management
            of, 35
        incidence, 29–30

management of, 32–35
    overview, 29–30
    recognition and
        detection of
        toxicity, 30–31
    polypharmacy, acute side
        effects of, 128
    serotonin syndrome and,
        159
Opisthotonos, 4
Overt Agitation Severity
    Scale, 16
Oxazepam, risk of seizures
    with, 151
Oxcarbazepine
    Brugada syndrome and,
        41
    as cause of SIADH or
        hyponatremia,
        83, 85, 88
    hepatotoxicity and, 67
    during pregnancy, 138
Oxycodone, combined with
    opioids, 31
Oxygen
    for management of acute
        dystonia, 7
    for management of
        coronary vasospasm,
        48
Oxymetazoline, hypertensive
    crisis and, 77

Paliperidone
    acute dystonia and, 4
    overdose of, 121
Parkinsonism, 5
Paroxetine
    AV block and, 44
    as cause of SIADH or
        hyponatremia, 84
    discontinuation of, 56
    ocular side effects of, 101
    during pregnancy, 136
Perphenazine, hepatotoxicity
    and, 66

Persistent postwithdrawal
    disorder
  anticonvulsants and, 56
  antipsychotic medications
    and, 52
  benzodiazepines and, 58
  description of, 51–52
  Z-drugs and, 58
Persistent pulmonary
    hypertension of the
    newborn (PPHN), 136
Pharyngeal spasms, 4
Phenelzine
  hepatotoxicity and, 65
  hypertensive crisis and, 75
  NMS and, 93
Phenothiazines
  ocular side effects of, 100
  oculogyric crisis and, 105
  pigmentary cataract
    deposits and, 106
  pigmentary retinal
    deposits and, 107
  TdP and, 40
Phentermine, hypertensive
    crisis and, 77
Phenylephrine, hypertensive
    crisis and, 77
Phenytoin, agranulocytosis
    and, 23
Phosphodiesterase inhibitors
  visual disturbances related
    to, 107–108
  assessment of, 108
  culprit medications,
    107
  description of, 107
  follow-up management
    of, 108
  management of, 108
  recognition and
    detection of, 107
Physostigmine
  for management of
    antipsychotic
    overdose, 120, 121

for treatment of
    antimuscarinic
    toxicity, 123
Pigmentary cataract deposits
  assessment of, 106
  culprit medications, 106
  description of, 105
  follow-up management of,
    106
  management of, 106
  recognition and detection
    of, 106
Pigmentary retinal deposits
  assessment of, 107
  culprit medications, 107
  description of, 106
  follow-up management of,
    107
  management of, 107
  recognition and detection
    of, 106
Pimozide, acute dystonia
    and, 3
Pittsburgh Agitation Scale, 16
Polycyclic aromatic
    hydrocarbons, nicotine
    and, 173
Polypharmacy, acute side
    effects of
  adverse drug events, 125
  assessment of, 129
  culprit medications,
    126–129
    anticholinergics,
      126–127
    antipsychotics, 128–129
    benzodiazepines,
      127–128
    opioids and narcotic
      analgesics, 128
  definition of, 125, 131
  follow-up management of,
    130
  management of, 129–130,
    131
  overview, 125

during pregnancy, 144
recognition and detection
of, 126
PPHN (persistent pulmonary
hypertension of the
newborn), 136
Pramipexole
for treatment of bipolar
depression, 14
for treatment of major
depressive disorder,
14
Pregabalin, hepatotoxicity
and, 68
Pregnancy, use of
psychotropic medication
during
assessment of, 140
culprit medications,
136–140
antipsychotics, 139
atomoxetine, 139
benzodiazepines,
139–140
bupropion, 137
carbamazepine, 138
lamotrigine, 138
lithium, 137–138
mirtazapine, 137
oxcarbazepine, 138
psychostimulants, 139
selective serotonin
reuptake
inhibitors, 136
serotonin-
norepinephrine
reuptake
inhibitors, 137
topiramate, 138
trazodone, 137
tricyclic antidepressants,
137
valproic acid, 138
follow-up management of,
142–143
lamotrigine, 142

lithium, 142–143
SSRIs, 142
illness
difficult cases, 141–142
mild, 141
moderate to severe, 141
lactation and, 143
management of, 140
miscarriage, 136
overview, 135
patient education and
counseling, 141
psychiatric illness, 143–144
recognition and detection
of, 136
Pregnancy and Lactation
Labeling Rule, 135
Primidone, agranulocytosis
and, 23
Prochlorperazine
agranulocytosis and, 23
hepatotoxicity and, 66
TD and, 184
Promazine, agranulocytosis
and, 23
Propranolol
AV block and, 44
for management of
serotonin syndrome,
163
Pseudodystonia, 5
Pseudoephedrine,
hypertensive crisis and,
77
Pseudomacroglossia, 4
Psilocybin (magic
mushrooms), addiction
to, 175
Psychedelics, addiction to
assessment of, 175
management of, 176
recognition and detection
of, 175
Psychoeducation
about agranulocytosis, 26
for seizures, 154

Psychogenic dystonia, 5
Psychogenic polydipsia
    as cause of SIADH or
        hyponatremia,
        85–86, 89
    prevalence of, 85
    treatment of, 87
Psychomotor agitation, 11.
        See also Agitation
    agitation and, 13
    description of, 18
    rating scales of, 16
    treatment for, 17
    underlying cause of, 18
Psychostimulants, during
        pregnancy, 139
Psychotherapy, for treatment
        of hyponatremia, 87
Psychotropic medications.
        See also Agranulocytosis,
        with clozapine and
        other psychotropic
        medications; Pregnancy,
        use of psychotropic
        medication during
    abrupt discontinuation of,
        144
    acute dystonia and, 8
    addiction to, 177
        follow-up management
            of, 176
    discontinuation of
        antidepressants, 55–57
        antipsychotic
            medications,
            52–53
        benzodiazepines and Z-
            drugs, 57–59
        collaborate effort with,
            60
        mood stabilizers, 53–55
        overview, 51–52
        withdrawal symptoms
            of, 60
    hepatotoxicity and
        assessment of, 68–69

    follow-up management
        of, 70–71
    management of, 70
    hepatotoxicity of
        assessment of, 68–69
        culprit medications,
            64–68
        antidepressants,
            64–65
        antipsychotics, 66–67
        benzodiazepines, 68
        mood stabilizers,
            67–68
        nonbenzodiazepine
            receptor
            agonists, 68
        follow-up management
            of, 70–75
        management of, 70
        overview, 63
        recognition and
            detection of, 64
    infant exposure to, 144
    life-threatening cardiac
            adverse events and,
            49
    ocular side effects of,
            99–109
        abnormal pigmentation
            of external ocular
            structures,
            99–100
        assessment of, 100
        culprit medications,
            100
        follow-up
            management
            of, 100
        management of,
            100
        recognition and
            detection of,
            99–100
    acute angle-closure
            glaucoma,
            100–102

assessment of,
101–102
culprit medications,
101
description of,
100–101
follow-up
management
of, 102
management of, 102
recognition and
detection of,
101
routine evaluation
with eye
specialist, 102
eye movement
abnormalities not
associated with
oculogyric crisis,
102–103
assessment of, 103
culprit medications,
103
follow-up
management
of, 103
management of, 103
mechanism of, 102
recognition and
detection of,
102–103
mydriasis and
cycloplegia
assessment of, 104
culprit medications,
104
description of,
103–104
follow-up
management
of, 104
management of, 104
recognition and
detection of,
104

oculogyric crisis,
104–105
assessment of, 105
culprit medications,
105
follow-up
management
of, 105
management of, 105
recognition and
detection of,
105
overview, 99
pigmentary cataract
deposits, 105–106
assessment of, 106
culprit medications,
106
follow-up
management
of, 106
management of, 106
recognition and
detection of,
106
pigmentary retinal
deposits, 106–107
assessment of, 107
culprit medications,
107
description of, 106
follow-up
management
of, 107
management of, 107
recognition and
detection of,
106
visual disturbances re-
lated to phospho-
diesterase
inhibitors,
107–108
assessment of, 108
culprit medications,
107

Psychotropic medications
  (continued)
  ocular side effects of
      (continued)
    visual disturbances
        related to
        phosphodiesterase
        inhibitors
        (continued)
      description of, 107
      follow-up
          management
          of, 108
      management of, 108
      recognition and
          detection of,
          107
  overdoses of, 111–124
    antidepressants,
        116–117
      tricyclic, 112–114
    antipsychotics, 119–122
      atypical, 120–122
      typical, 119–120
    lithium, 117–118
    overview, 111
    psychiatric consultation
        of patients, 118
    selective serotonin
        reuptake
        inhibitors, 114–115
    serotonin-
        norepinephrine
        reuptake
        inhibitors,
        115–116
    supportive care and, 122
    tricyclic antidepressants,
        112–114
  overview, xv–xvi
  persistent postwithdrawal
      disorder, 51–52
  during pregnancy, 140
  rebound symptoms, 51
  toxicity from, 122
  withdrawal symptoms, 51

Quetiapine
  acute dystonia and, 4
  hepatotoxicity and,
      66–67
  risk of seizures with, 150
Quinolinones, toxicity from,
    121

Rebound symptoms
  anticonvulsants and, 56
  antipsychotic medications
      and, 52
  benzodiazepines and, 58
  description of, 51
  Z-drugs and, 58
Repetitive transcranial
    magnetic stimulation
    (rTMS)
  risk of seizures with, 152
  TD and, 189
Reserpine, TD and, 189
Restless legs syndrome
    (RLS), antipsychotic
    medications and, 13
Retina. See Pigmentary
    retinal deposits
Reversible inhibitors of
    MAO-A (RIMAs), 76
Richmond Agitation-
    Sedation Scale, 16
RIMAs (reversible inhibitors
    of MAO-A), 76
Risperidone
  acute dystonia and, 4
  overdose of, 121
  oculogyric crisis and, 105
Ritonavir, serotonin
    syndrome and, 159
Rivastigmine, hepatotoxicity
    and, 68
RLS (restless legs syndrome),
    antipsychotic
    medications and, 13
rTMS. See Repetitive
    transcranial magnetic
    stimulation

Schooler-Kane criteria, 186
Second-generation agents
      (SGAs)
   agitation and, 12–13
   hepatotoxicity and, 66
   polypharmacy, acute side
         effects of, 129
Second-generation
      antipsychotics (SGAs),
      52
Seizures
   assessment of, 152
   culprit medications
      antidepressants,
            149–150
      antipsychotics, 150–151
      anxiolytics, 151
      mood stabilizers, 150
      overview, 149
      rTMS and psychoactive
            medications, 152
      stimulants, 151
   drop attacks, 148
   EEG for, 153
   epileptic, 147
   epileptiform, 147–148
   ethanol and, 168
   follow-up management of,
         153–154
   grand mal, 147
   GTCS, 147
   management of, 152–153
   overview, 147–148
   prolonged, 154
   rapid response team and,
         152–153
   recognition and detection,
         148–149
      generalized seizure
            types, 148
      GTCS, 148
      nonepileptiform
            seizures, 148–149
      simple and complex
            partial seizure,
            148

   risks for, 154
   status epilepticus, 153
   toxicity-induced, 120, 121
Selective serotonin reuptake
      inhibitors (SSRIs)
   agitation and, 11–12
   as cause of SIADH or
         hyponatremia, 83
   discontinuation of, 55–57
   ethanol and, 168
   follow-up management of
         infant exposure to,
         142
   hepatotoxicity and, 65
   NMS and, 93
   ocular side effects of, 101
   overdose of
      assessment of, 114
      follow-up management
            of, 115
      management of, 115
      recognition and
            detection of, 114
   during pregnancy, 136
   serotonin syndrome and,
         158, 159
Selegiline
   hepatotoxicity and, 64, 65
   hypertensive crisis and, 75
   TD and, 189
Serotonin, toxicity, 116
Serotonin-norepinephrine
      reuptake inhibitors
      (SNRIs)
   agitation and, 11–12
   agranulocytosis and, 23
   as cause of SIADH or
         hyponatremia, 83
   discontinuation of, 55–57
   overdose of
      assessment of, 115
      follow-up management
            of, 116
      management of, 115–116
      recognition and
            detection of, 115

Serotonin-norepinephrine
reuptake inhibitors
(SNRIs) *(continued)*
during pregnancy, 137
risk of seizures with,
149–150
serotonin syndrome and,
159
Serotonin syndrome, 12, 119
assessment of, 159–162
causes of, 165
characterization of, 164
culprit medications,
158–159
diagnosis of, 171
follow-up management of,
164
incidence of, 157
management of, 162–164,
165
overview, 157–158
patient-related causes of,
157–158
prognosis of, 164
psychedelics and, 175
recognition and detection
of, 158
SSRIs and, 158
stimulants and, 170
symptoms of, 158
treatment as a medical
emergency, 172
Sertraline
agranulocytosis and, 23
ethanol and, 168
hepatotoxicity and, 64
during pregnancy, 136
serotonin syndrome and,
159
SGAs. *See* Second-generation
agents; Second-
generation antipsychotics
SIADH (syndrome of
inappropriate
antidiuretic hormone
secretion), 81

Sick sinus syndrome (sinus
node dysfunction)
assessment of, 43
culprit medication, 43
description of, 42
follow-up management of,
43
management of, 43
recognition and detection
of, 42
Sildenafil, visual
disturbances related to,
107–108
SILENT (syndrome of
irreversible lithium-
effectuated
neurotoxicity), 117
Sinus node dysfunction.
See Sick sinus syndrome
Sleep-related activities,
nonbenzodiazepines
and, 14
SNRIs. *See* Serotonin-
norepinephrine
reuptake inhibitors
Sodium, 82–83. *See also*
Hyponatremia
baseline, 88
Sodium channel blockers,
ventricular conduction
delay and, 45
SSRIs. *See* Selective serotonin
reuptake inhibitors
Status epilepticus, 153
Steatosis, 63
Steroids, risk of seizures
with, 152
Stimulants
addiction to, 177
assessment of, 171
management of,
171–172
recognition and
detection of,
170–171
cannabis and, 172–173

death from, 171
ethanol and, 169
hypertensive crisis and, 77
risk of seizures with, 151,
152
St. John's wort, serotonin
syndrome and, 159
Substance use.
See also Addiction
serotonin syndrome and,
160
Succinylcholine, for
management of
serotonin syndrome, 164
Sudden death, 4
acute dystonia and, 4
Sulpiride, TD and, 189
Sympathomimetics, 79
hypertensive crisis and, 77
Syndrome malin des
neuroleptiques.
See Neuroleptic
malignant syndrome
Syndrome of inappropriate
antidiuretic hormone
secretion (SIADH), 81
Syndrome of irreversible
lithium-effectuated
neurotoxicity (SILENT),
117

Tacrine, hepatotoxicity and,
68
Tadalafil, visual disturbances
related to, 107–108
Tardive akathisia, 53
agitation and, 12–13
Tardive dyskinesia (TD), 53
antipsychotic drugs and,
190
assessment of, 185
culprit medications,
184–185
description of, 181
differential diagnosis of,
183

DSM-5-TR description of,
184
DSM-5-TR diagnosis of,
185
pathophysiology of, 181
prevalence of, 181–182
recognition and detection
of, 184
relapse of, 189
risk factors for, 182–183
treatment of, 183–184, 190
Tardive dystonia, 5
TCAs. *See* Tricyclic
antidepressants
TD. *See* Tardive dyskinesia
TdP. *See* Torsades de pointes
Temporal lobe epilepsies, 5
Δ-9-Tetrahydrocannabinol (Δ-
9-THC), 172
Δ-9-THC (Δ-9-
tetrahydrocannabinol),
172
Thiamine, TD and, 189
Thiazides, as cause of SIADH
or hyponatremia, 83
Thiazine diuretics, 12
Thiopropazate, TD and, 189
Thioridazine
agranulocytosis and, 23
hepatotoxicity and, 66
ocular side effects of, 100
pigmentary cataract
deposits and, 106
pigmentary retinal
deposits and, 107
polypharmacy, acute side
effects of, 129
risk of seizures with, 150
TdP and, 40
Topiramate
as cause of SIADH or
hyponatremia, 85
hepatotoxicity and, 66–67
oculogyric crisis and,
105
during pregnancy, 138

Torsades de pointes (TdP)
  assessment of, 40
  culprit medications, 40
  description of, 39
  management of, 40–41
  recognition and detection
    of, 40
Torticollis, 4
Tortipelvic crisis, 4
Toxicity. *See also* Death
  acute-on-chronic, 117
  from antidepressants,
    174
  from antipsychotics, 122
  idiosyncratic, 63
  -induced seizures, 120
  from lithium, 14, 15, 117,
    122
  nicotine and, 174, 175
  opioid-benzodiazepines
    and, 36
  from overdoses of
    psychotropic
    medications, 111
  from psychotropic
    medications, 122
  from quinolinones, 121
  recognition and detection
    of, 30–31
  with sertraline, 65
  stimulants and, 171–172
Toxidromes, 162, 164, 165. *See
  also* Serotonin syndrome
Tramadol, as cause of SIADH
  or hyponatremia, 83
Tranylcypromine
  agranulocytosis and, 23
  hepatotoxicity and, 65
  hypertensive crisis and, 75
Trazodone
  discontinuation of, 55
  hepatotoxicity and, 64
  overdose of, 116
  during pregnancy, 137
  serotonin syndrome and,
    159

Tricyclic antidepressants
    (TCAs)
  agitation and, 12
  agranulocytosis and, 23
  anticholinergic effects and,
    126–127
  AV block and, 44
  Brugada syndrome and, 41
  as cause of SIADH or
    hyponatremia, 83
  ethanol and, 168
  hepatotoxicity and, 65
  myocarditis and, 46
  NMS and, 93
  ocular side effects of, 101
  overdose of
    assessment of, 113
    follow-up management
      of, 114
    management of,
      113–114
    recognition and
      detection of, 112
  during pregnancy, 137
  psychedelics and, 175
  risk of seizures with, 149,
    152
  serotonin syndrome and,
    159
  stimulants and, 170
  TdP and, 40
  ventricular conduction
    delay and, 45
Trifluoperazine
  Brugada syndrome and,
    41
  hepatotoxicity and, 66
Trimethadione,
    agranulocytosis and, 23
Triptans, serotonin syndrome
    and, 159
Trismus, 4
L-Tryptophan, serotonin
    syndrome and, 159
Tyramine, dietary, 76, 79
  ethanol and, 168

Urine
    drug screening and, 171
    retention of, 162
    serotonin syndrome and,
        161
Urological medications,
    anticholinergic effects
    and, 127
U.S. FDA Clozapine Risk
    Evaluation and
    Mitigation Strategy
    program, 26, 27

Valbenazine
    for management of
        antipsychotic
        medications, 53
    TD and, 187, 188–189
Valproate
    agitation and, 13–14
    as cause of SIADH or
        hyponatremia, 85
    discontinuation of, 54
    hepatotoxicity and, 67
Valproic acid
    NMS and, 93
    overdose of, 111
    during pregnancy, 138, 142
Vardenafil, visual disturbances
    related to, 107–108
Vasodilators, for
    management of
    coronary vasospasm, 48
Vecuronium, for
    management of
    serotonin syndrome, 164
Venlafaxine
    ethanol and, 168
    hepatotoxicity and, 64
    during pregnancy, 137
Ventricular conduction delay
    assessment of, 45
    culprit medications, 45
    description of, 45
    follow-up management of,
        45

management of, 45
recognition and detection
    of, 45
Vesicular monoamine
    transporter type 2
    (VMAT2) inhibitors, 53
    NMS and, 93
    TD and, 187, 191
Vilazodone
    discontinuation of, 55
    risk of seizures with,
        150
Vision. See also Eyes;
        Pigmentary retinal
        deposits
    blue tinge, 107
    blurry, 107, 127
    double, 102–103
    nighttime, 106
    visual disturbances related
        to phosphodiesterase
        inhibitors, 107–108
Vitamin B_6, TD and, 189
Vitamin E, TD and, 189
VMAT2. See Vesicular
        monoamine transporter
        type 2 inhibitors
Vortioxetine, discontinuation
        of, 55

Wilson's disease, 5
Withdrawal symptoms
    antipsychotic medications
        and, 52
    description of, 51
Women. See also Pregnancy,
        use of psychotropic
        medication during
    depression and anxiety in,
        135
    with mental illness during
        pregnancy, 144
    reproductive safety data
        for, 144
    SIADH and, 81
    with TD, 182–183

Young Mania Rating Scale, 16

Zaleplon, combined with
    opioids, 31
Z-drugs
    combined with opioids, 31
    discontinuation of, 57–59
        assessment of, 58
        follow-up management
            of, 59
        management of, 58–59
        recognition and
            detection of, 57–58
            persistent postwith-
                drawal disor-
                der, 58

rebound symptoms,
    58
withdrawal
    symptoms,
    57–58
Ziprasidone
    acute dystonia and, 4
    overdose of, 121
    risk of seizures with, 150
    TdP and, 40
Zolpidem, combined with
    opioids, 31
Zopiclone, combined with
    opioids, 31